This book was published by the Kolbe Center for the Study of Creation

952 Kelly Rd. Mt. Jackson, VA 22842

For more information or to order additional copies of this book please go to:

www.kolbecenter.org

ISBN: 978-0-9715691-5-7

First Printing: December 12, 2020

**IMPRIMATUR**

✠ Rt. Rev. Dr. Joseph Eciru Oliarch
Bishop of Soroti Catholic Diocese
01 March 2021

In grateful memory of Fr. Thomas Hickey,

who taught me how to be a better Catholic

and a better scientist

# Contents

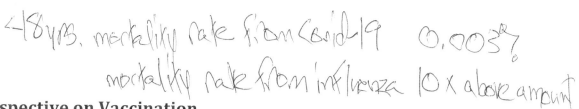

*-18yrs, mortality rate from Covid-19   0.003%*
*mortality rate from influenza 10x above amount*

# A Catholic Perspective on Vaccination

*Any preventive, diagnostic and therapeutic medical intervention is only to be carried out with the prior, free and informed consent of the person concerned, based on adequate information. The consent should, where appropriate, be express and may be withdrawn by the person concerned at any time and for any reason without disadvantage or prejudice.*
*-- Universal Declaration on Bioethics and Human Rights[1]*

There is much controversy surrounding the subject of vaccinating children and infants against what are generally termed "preventable childhood diseases." On the one hand, supporters of vaccination urge it not only as a medical necessity for the individuals vaccinated, but as an ethical duty for the common good of society (both here and abroad). On the other hand, hundreds of thousands of individuals report what are known as "adverse reactions" to vaccines, stories that remain largely anecdotal in their nature but are gravely consequential if true. The vaccine supporters urge us to dismiss such stories on the grounds that the scientific evidence suggests that vaccines are safe and effective, while the vaccine opponents argue that the very cases they are reporting (along with additional information about the toxicity of individual vaccine components) are the scientific evidence needed to invalidate the claims of both safety and efficacy. Both sides are looking at what amounts to the same evidence, much as in the debate over the theory of evolution, but they are coming to startlingly different conclusions.

Meanwhile, there is also confusion among Catholics regarding whether it is morally permissible to refuse vaccination (in light of concerns over compromising herd immunity* in the population) but also about whether it is morally permissible to receive vaccination (in light of the use of aborted fetal cells in the development of certain vaccines).

In order to provide a coherent answer to the controversy surrounding vaccination, it is imperative to examine the issue from multiple angles, including the history of vaccination, the biology of the immune system and the induction of the vaccine response, the safety of vaccines in light of our understanding of these biological principles, the morality of vaccination (particularly as a pro-life issue, which relates to both the concept of herd immunity and to the use of aborted fetal cells), and the reasonable alternatives to mass vaccination. An additional facet of the discussion that will be unique to this work is a brief examination of the relationship between the ideology behind vaccination and the pervasive paradigm of evolution theory as it affects modern medicine. All of these topics will be unpacked in the pages that follow.

---

[1] United Nations Educational, Scientific, and Cultural Organization (UNESCO). Universal Declaration on Bioethics and Human Rights. 19 Oct 2005. http://portal.unesco.org/en/ev.php-URL_ID=31058&URL_DO=DO_TOPIC&URL_SECTION=201.html Accessed 26 Oct 2019.

* Briefly explained, herd immunity is the idea that if enough individuals in a group are immune to a disease, the disease will not spread through the group (whether it be a local population, a nation, or the global population) because the likelihood of an infected individual coming into contact with a susceptible individual will be quite low. The disease would be transmitted only inefficiently, if at all, and the possibility of an epidemic would be curtailed. Herd immunity is ultimately the goal of mass vaccination programs and vaccination advocates based their argument on the idea that achieving herd immunity is consistent with the common good.

# A Brief History of Vaccination

*Amateur critics often like to dismiss anecdotes as 'unscientific,' but this is wrong: anecdotes are weaker evidence than trials, but they are not without value, and are often the first sign of a problem.*
*-- Dr. Ben Goldacre[2]*

It is a good practice to establish one's credentials at the outset of an argument, so I will begin with a brief introduction of my own history with the vaccine controversy, which began in the late 1990s. As a high school biology student, I was fascinated by both immunology and genetics, and very interested in researching genetic modification of fruiting plants to deliver vaccines. The idea particularly appealed to me as it would have been a much more reasonable method for storing and transporting life-saving doses of medication in Third World countries. Ultimately, the technology was abandoned due to an inability to standardize the dosages of vaccine antigen* in the fruits, but that did not dampen my enthusiasm for either vaccines or genetics. It was around this time that I also became acquainted with the work of Children of God for Life, a Catholic organization that promotes awareness of the immoral use of aborted fetal tissue in vaccines.[3] My interest in plant-based vaccines was in large part motivated by a desire to generate ethical alternatives to these unethical vaccines. I studied biology in college and applied to the Danforth Center (the major research institution investigating genetically engineered plant vaccines) but ended up working in genomics and later in education. I put the idea of vaccine development on the back burner and tried to find other ways to support the pro-life cause.

About six years later, the issue of vaccines resurfaced. I decided to return to graduate school for further studies in biology and was accepted into the Rao Laboratory at The Catholic University of America. It was here that I worked directly on research for an HIV vaccine. My corner of the project was primarily focused on finding molecular methods to target our novel vaccine delivery platform (which was a modified form of an *E. coli* virus) to interact directly with immune system cells. I ultimately resigned my position in the lab, and abandoned my pursuit of a PhD, when I learned that the vaccine antigens were being produced in a strain of aborted fetal cells (HEK-293). I continued to research HIV and vaccines even after leaving the lab, and while I do not agree with the ethical position the university ultimately took,* I am thankful for having had the experience of

---

[2] Goldacre B. *Bad Pharma*. New York: Faber and Faber, 2012, p. 87.

* An antigen is a molecular marker that allows a cell to be recognized by the immune system. Often it is a carbohydrate or protein, and because of its unique shape, it can serve as a "tag" to identify a particular kind of pathogen. The curious reader can find more information about antigens here:
https://medlineplus.gov/ency/article/002224.htm

[3] Children of God for Life. https://cogforlife.org/
Their vaccine chart (https://cogforlife.org/wp-content/uploads/vaccineListOrigFormat.pdf) gives an excellent quick reference for unethical vaccines and any alternatives that are available.

* In the spring of 2011, CUA officials ruled that although the procurement of aborted fetal cells was no longer going to be permitted, the labs that had these cells on hand could use them until they ran out. It is unlikely that the decision makers were aware that a large stock of HEK-293 cells were being kept in freezers, and that these cells could be sub-cultured for many years before the labs would have to order new cells. If the policy has changed in the intervening years, it is only to have become less restrictive: the most recent paper published by the Rao Lab (April 2020) lists HEK-293 cells in the materials and methods section. See: Zhu, J., Tao, P., Mahalingam, M. and Rao, V. (2020). Preparation of a Bacteriophage T4-based Prokaryotic-eukaryotic Hybrid Viral Vector for Delivery of Large Cargos of Genes and Proteins into Human Cells. *Bio-protocol* 10(7): e3573. doi: 10.21769/BioProtoc.3573.

spending nearly a year in the quest to create a new vaccine. It has given me an insight into this complex subject that has proven invaluable.

At this point, I will turn from this personal history to a more general history of vaccination. This topic is particularly important because much of the actual history of vaccination is never taught in schools, and the bias with which much of the information is presented invariably confuses the issue.

## Edward Jenner and the Smallpox Vaccine

If you have been exposed to any information about the development of vaccination in a high school biology course or through reading a popular scientific history, you have surely heard the name of Edward Jenner. In popular culture, Jenner is celebrated and surrounded with an almost savior-like halo for having made the most important discovery in the annals of modern medicine.[4] The depth of the emotional attachment to the idea of "saving vaccines" is so deep in our culture that our local libraries even have children's books on the shelves that bear titles such as *You Wouldn't Want to Live Without Vaccinations!*.[5] While the popular halo is appealing, as there is a human tendency to idolize important historical figures, it is helpful to look behind the curtain to observe the actual events that accompanied the introduction and widespread dissemination of vaccination.

Smallpox was a serious disease in the 1800s, claiming approximately 15 million lives in Europe every 25 years during that century.[6] Because of the severity of the disease, individuals were open to methods that promised protection, even if they caused other, potentially serious, health problems. In Jenner's day, a protective practice called variolation was in vogue in England. This involved taking dried scabs from smallpox victims and grinding them into a preparation that a healthy individual would then inhale.[7] Alternatively, the matter could be scratched into the surface of a person's arm.[8] The practice was somewhat grotesque and, as an unfortunate side effect, could result in the patient contracting smallpox, and even dying from the disease. It also often started actual outbreaks of smallpox as the virus spread to the contacts of the patient.[9] According to some estimates:

> [I]n the 38 years preceding the start of inoculation [variolation through scratching material into the arm] in 1721, deaths from smallpox relative to the number born was 90 per 1,000, and relative to the number of burials 64 per 1000. In the 38 years after the start of inoculation, deaths from smallpox relative to the number born increased to 127 per 1000 (a 41 percent increase) and relative to the number of burials 81 per 1,000 (a 27 percent increase).[10]

---

[4] NOVA. *Vaccines: Calling the Shots*, 2014. DVD. Boston: PBS.

[5] Rooney A. *You Wouldn't Want to Live Without Vaccinations*. Brighton, UK: The Salariya Book Company, 2015.

[6] Diodati CJM. *Immunization: History, Ethics, Law and Health*. Ontario, CN: Integral Aspects Incorporated, 1999, p. 4.

[7] Rooney A. *You Wouldn't Want to Live Without Vaccinations*. Brighton, UK: The Salariya Book Company, 2015.

[8] Humphries S and Bystrianyk R. *Dissolving Illusions*. Printed by author. 2015, p 66-67.

[9] Ibid, p. 88-94.

[10] Ibid, p. 62. cf. "The Practice of Inoculation Truly Stated," *The Gentleman's Magazine and Historical Chronicle*, vol. 34, 1764, p. 333.

The ineffectiveness of variolation led enterprising individuals to look for an alternative method of protection from "the pox." The popular form of the story goes that Edward Jenner noticed that dairy maids, who are often infected with cowpox from the cows they milk, were generally protected from smallpox. He wondered whether inoculating someone with cowpox would be protective against the dreaded smallpox. In reality, Jenner was not the first to notice this phenomenon, nor the first to test it. A farmer named Benjamin Jesty tried deliberately infecting his wife and two sons with cowpox 22 years before Jenner performed his experiment with his own son and a neighbor boy, James Phipps, in 1796.[11]

Unlike Jesty, Jenner did not obtain his disease material directly from a cow, but from pustules on the hand of a dairy maid (Sarah Nelmes) that he presumed were cowpox.[*] He inoculated both boys, and later deliberately exposed Phipps to smallpox by introducing smallpox-infected serum directly into the boy's arm through two cuts.[12] Phipps did not develop smallpox, and according to most histories available today, the development was hailed as a medical breakthrough. Vaccination was inaugurated.

A few key details are left out of this narrative, however. In 1798, Jenner developed a new vaccine that combined disease matter from "horse grease"[•] with the cowpox material and promoted it as more effective than his original serum. However, experiments showed that the new treatment was not very effective at all, and Jenner returned to promoting his original cowpox concoction.[13] The public was also uncomfortable with being infected with disease material that originated in animals, which helped to squelch Jenner's new vaccine, but also led to smallpox vaccine material being transferred between human patients who were inoculated. A pox pustule on one vaccinated patient would be opened, and the material scratched into the arm of another patient to vaccinate him against the disease.[14] This led to the transmission of a number of serious blood-borne diseases through vaccination, including tuberculosis, smallpox, and syphilis. After mandatory inoculation campaigns were instituted in the UK, the rate of deaths of infants from syphilis doubled in one year.[15] Both Jenner's son and James Phipps died in their early 20s from tuberculosis,[16] which was likely transmitted to them through Jenner's initial vaccination.

Almost from the beginning, Jenner's claims of lifelong immunity were challenged by medical professionals. Within only a few years, estimates of immune persistence suggested that his vaccine provided only 1-10 years of protection against smallpox. In 1911, one practitioner went so far as

---

[11] Ibid, p. 62- 65.

[*] No serological testing was done to confirm the nature of the disease material, and this lack of testing remained a problem throughout the history of smallpox vaccination. Often physicians themselves did not know the real nature of the infectious material they were injecting – whether it was smallpox, cowpox, rabbit-pox, mule-pox, or pox from some other species, or whether it was contaminated with other communicable diseases like syphilis or hoof-and-mouth. (*See* Humphries and Bystrianyk, 2015, p 65-69.)

[12] Diodati CJM. *Immunization: History, Ethics, Law and Health.* Ontario, CN: Integral Aspects Incorporated, 1999, p. 5.

[•] This condition was commonly found in cart horses kept in unsanitary conditions, and was often confused with horse pox. (See Diodati, 1999, p. 23, n 16.)

[13] Ibid.

[14] Humphries S and Bystrianyk R. *Dissolving Illusions.* Printed by author. 2015, p. 66-67.

[15] Hail AR. *The Medical Voodoo.* Gotham House, New York. 1935, p 66. *See* Diodati, 1999, p. 22.

[16] Diodati CJM. *Immunization: History, Ethics, Law and Health.* Ontario, CN: Integral Aspects Incorporated, 1999, p. 22-23.

to recommend yearly revaccination for smallpox, much as is now recommended for the flu.[17] However, continual revaccination led to smallpox epidemics in England and in other areas of Europe.[18] When the vaccine began to be manufactured on a larger scale, contamination with hoof-and-mouth disease proved debilitating or even fatal in some individuals receiving the vaccine.[19] Despite all of these problems, mandatory vaccination laws forced parents to pay a fine or go to prison for refusing to vaccinate their children, even if one member in the family had already experienced a severe or life-threatening reaction to the smallpox vaccine.[20]

This is only a small piece of the picture of the advent of vaccination, and there is much more that could be said about the smallpox vaccine and other vaccines. For a more detailed account of the history of vaccination, including a thorough treatment of the history of polio and measles vaccines, I refer the reader to the book *Dissolving Illusions* by Dr. Suzanne Humphries, MD and Roman Bystrianyk. They have done more work to illuminate the subject than I possibly could here, and their book is extremely well referenced with many primary sources from medical journals of the time periods they describe.

## *Vaccination, or Sanitation?*

Another tremendous service that these two authors have done to the debate about vaccination is to provide a tremendous amount of evidence that death rates in the major vaccine-preventable diseases were dropping long before the introduction of the vaccines.[21] The high mortality rates of disease in the pre-vaccination era can be rightly attributed to the following factors:

- Poor housing: At the time of industrialization, many individuals moved from rural areas into cities. The influx of people was too overwhelming to be accommodated by current housing structures, and so individuals were forced to share crowded spaces in tenement houses. In some cases, small families shared spaces as large as a modern walk-in closet.[22]

- Poor sanitation: Crowded housing brought with it poor waste removal. Sometimes a whole building would be privy to a single outhouse; at other times, waste was deposited directly into alleys. This had a profoundly negative impact on the quality of available water, as waste and even sewage was deposited in streams that served as the primary water source for an area. Ventilation in the tenement buildings was also often poor.[23]

- Animals: Not only were domestic animals living in close quarters with men in the crowded tenement housing, but feral animals (mainly rats, insects, and dogs) also abounded. The rats sometimes even attacked humans.[24]

---

[17] Humphries S and Bystrianyk R. *Dissolving Illusions*. Printed by author. 2015, p 63-64.
[18] Ibid, p. 59-95.
[19] Ibid, p. 96-112.
[20] Ibid, p. 117.
[21] Ibid, p. 196-201.
[22] Ibid, p. 1-9.
[23] Ibid, p. 1-11.
[24] Ibid, p. 12-14.

- Poor nutrition: Diseased animals were often slaughtered and their meat was marketed as sausages or pies. The few vegetables that could be obtained in the city were often rotten. Milk came from cows that were kept in unsanitary conditions, and its poor quality was held responsible for sickness and even death among large numbers of children.[25]

- Extreme working conditions: Child labor was permitted at this time, and many children worked long hours (up to 14-15 hours per day) at back-breakingly difficult tasks. This led not only to on-the-job mortality (such as children being run over by carts or badly burned when operating furnaces) but also to high mortality rates from being constantly overworked and exhausted. Women fared little better at this time, often working up to 100 hours per week.[26]

- Loss of care from mothers: Childbed fever was rampant, with as many as 50% of mothers being lost during childbirth at particularly disreputable hospitals. Mothers who survived might work long hours and be often away from their small children. Both of these factors likely contributed to higher-than-normal infant and childhood mortality, as infants were less likely to be breast-fed and children were less likely to receive adequate maternal care.[27]

Most of these deplorable conditions were resolved or on their way to resolution by the early 20th century, before the introduction of most vaccines.[28] Indeed, smallpox itself seemed to wane in its infectivity, and epidemics were finally contained by quarantine and sanitation (including in populations that were not vaccinated at all).[29] Lending even more credence to the case that it was sanitation and quality of life, rather than vaccination, that decreased disease mortality is the fact that diseases such as plague, cholera, and typhus fever had also receded into the past as scourges of society by the early 20th century.[30] There may have been no need to attempt to modify the immune system by introducing disease material into healthy individuals. However, since vaccination has become the norm rather than the exception, the next area to be explored on this topic is the biology of vaccination.

*Who gets TB odds from it? Another example, even today...*

[25] Ibid, p. 14-17.
[26] Ibid, p. 18-30.
[27] Ibid, p. 31, 53-58.
[28] Ibid.
[29] Ibid, p. 124-221.
[30] Anderson HB. *State Medicine a Menace to Democracy*, 1920. p. 84.

# The Biology of Vaccination

*Currently available vaccines have largely been developed empirically,*
*with little or no understanding of how they activate the immune system.*
*-- Plotkin's Vaccines*[31]

The history of vaccination may be checkered, but what of its practice in modern days? At the time that Jenner introduced the concept of vaccination as a method of disease prevention, very little was known about the mechanism of the immune system and its vital operations within the body. Modern science in this area has advanced so rapidly that what I learned as an undergraduate in 2004 was obsolete when I attended graduated school in 2010-2012, and what I learned in graduate school has been replaced by an even more complex array of cellular and molecular players whose coordinated efforts defend the body against any foreign invader. When these invaders have the capability of causing disease, they are called *pathogens*. To have a clear understanding of the debate surrounding vaccination, it is important to understand some of the developments in our knowledge of the immune system and its interaction with pathogens.

In order to be reasonably concise, the following explanation of the immune system will be something of an abridged version and will provide an inadequate picture of the marvel of design in the human body. Nevertheless, it will provide an essential basis for the subsequent discussion. In order to fully understand the nature of vaccination, and make informed decisions about whether to use vaccines, it is necessary to understand some of the component parts of the immune system and how they work, as well as what happens when the immune system fails to work properly. The remainder of the chapter will be devoted to an explanation of the antibody hypothesis and its relation to vaccination, as well as the different types of vaccines and the different biological effects of each type.

## *The Biology of the Immune System*

The immune system is the most amorphous of the body's systems, consisting not only of organs, but of specific tissues within organs that properly belong to other body systems, and also of individual cells that are able to migrate throughout the body. Figure 1, which displays a condensed pictorial representation of the cellular players in the immune system, gives some indication of the incredible diversity of cells that constitute the immune system. Because of its disconnected and sometimes microscopic nature, it is no wonder that the study of the immune system is such a recently developed science.

The function of the immune system can be broadly characterized as giving the body the ability to distinguish between cells and extracellular components that <u>are</u> a normal part of the body and those that <u>are not</u> a normal part of the body (i.e. between "self" and "non-self"). Once this determination has been made, the second major function of the immune system comes into play – to seek and destroy anything that is non-self.

---

[31] Siegrist CA. Vaccine Immunology. In: Plotkin SA, Offit, PA, Orenstein WA, Edwards KM. *Plotkin's Vaccines, 7th ed.* Philadelphia: Elsevier, 2018, p. 16-34.

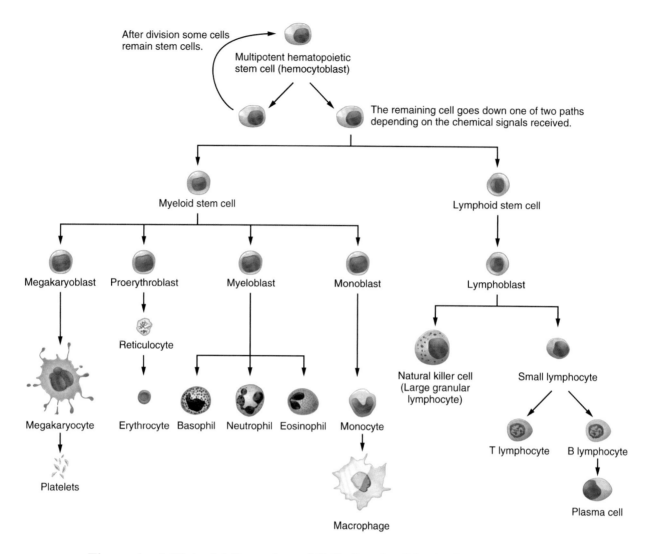

**Figure 1: A Pictorial Overview of Cells Involved in the Immune System**

The immune system does not stand alone, but depends on many other bodily systems to perform its functions. The first line of defense for the body against any pathogen is the simple barrier of the skin. Mucous membranes that line our mouth and respiratory cavities help trap any possible invaders. From the mouth and nasal cavities, mucous washes pathogens into the digestive tract where they are destroyed by the high acidity of the stomach. In addition, the circulatory and lymphatic systems are responsible for aiding in the transport of many immune cells throughout the body. Thus, we see that to truly understand the workings of the immune system requires an overarching understanding of human anatomy and physiology.

If the body's basic physical barriers are breached, the immune system's next defense is the inflammatory response. Inflammation is often associated with pain, redness, swelling, and heat; these symptoms are due to the cascade of signals that immune cells release when a pathogen is first detected. These signals result in dilation of blood vessels, which allow fluid and immune cells to escape into the affected area of the body. The extra fluid helps wash pathogens from the area, and the immune cells and their activities constitute the body's third line of defense. This is the facet of the immune system about which there is the most still to learn.

The body's circulating immune cells are collectively referred to as white blood cells. These cells are generally subdivided into two categories: *innate* and *adaptive*. Innate immune cells include macrophages, neutrophils, natural killer cells, and a number of other types of cells, which were for a long time thought to have a "non-specific" response to pathogens. A good analogy was to consider these cells as the "brute force" arm of the immune system – they would indiscriminately engulf and dissolve pathogens, sometimes dying themselves in the process, and create what amounted to massive cellular carnage while trying to keep the pathogen from reproducing at a rate that would overwhelm the body's defenses. The adaptive immune cells are primarily B cells and T cells. These cells were thought to be more refined in their approach, and only activate in response to one type of pathogen. The adaptive immune cells were long thought to be solely responsible for the function of *immunological memory*, or your body's ability to mount a more efficient response to a pathogen upon a second exposure.

The whole idea of vaccination is predicated upon an attempt to activate this memory function of the immune system – specifically, through the activation of the *antibody* response. B cells are a special class of adaptive immune cells that are responsible for producing small proteins called antibodies. Figure 2 gives an overview of how B cells are activated to produce these molecules. Antibodies are highly specific in their ability to bind to pathogens. A key will only open one lock, and a specific antibody molecule will only target one pathogen or one part of a pathogen[*] (usually called an *antigen*, which is short for "antibody generator"). There are several different types of antibodies with a variety of functions – there are antibodies that can "tag" the pathogen for elimination by other immune cells, prevent viruses from entering the cells they normally infect, neutralize toxins secreted by pathogens, and even cause bacterial cells to self-destruct by activating an internal signaling system that ends in cell death.[32] Antibodies were some of the first components of the immune system to be characterized, and their centrality to the idea of vaccination has remained unchallenged since their discovery.

It was originally thought that the innate immune cells only played a role in the immune system's initial, non-specific response to infection. If the innate cells failed to fully clear the pathogen from the body, they would activate the adaptive immune cells and their own role would be finished. Recent advances in immunology indicate, however, that such a simple two-step, one-way approach to understanding immune system activation is highly misleading. Dendritic cells that facilitate crosstalk between the adaptive and innate immune system, and fulfill other crucial functions in immune response, were discovered in the 1980s,[33] and have continued to change our understanding of the immune system up to the present day. We now know that the innate immune system does

---

[*] This is an oversimplification, as we now know that there is some cross-reactivity between similar pathogens. For example, if the body has a memory response to one strain of the flu, a similar strain may activate the memory response for the first flu. (See: Kelly H, Barry S, Laurie K, Mercer G. Seasonal influenza vaccination and the risk of infection with pandemic influenza: a possible illustration of nonspecific temporary immunity following infection. *Euro Surveill.* 2010; 15(47).) There may even be cross-reactivity across different genera of viruses.

[32] Murphy K, Travers P, Walport M. *Janeway's Immunobiology, 9th Ed.* New York and London: Garland Science, Taylor & Francis Group, 2017, p. 422-431.

[33] The Rockefeller University. "Discovery." 25 March 2015. http://lab.rockefeller.edu/steinman/dendritic_intro/discovery Accessed 20 April 2020.

not have a one-and-done role in the initial stages of infection, but can also be activated by the adaptive arm of the immune defenses.[34] The most recent research indicates that the innate immune system even functions in some type of immunological memory, often referred to as "trained immunity" to differentiate it from adaptive immunological memory.[35]

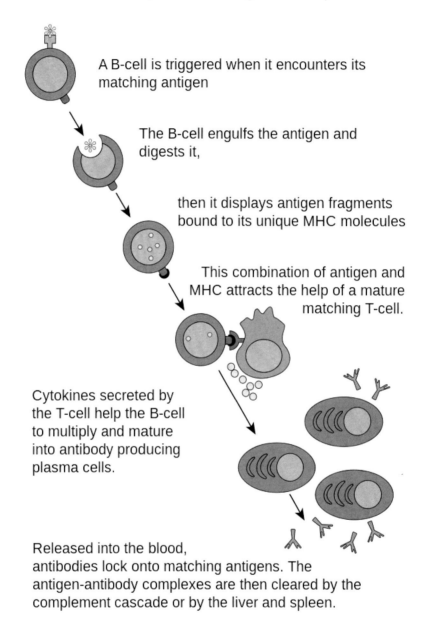

A B-cell is triggered when it encounters its matching antigen

The B-cell engulfs the antigen and digests it,

then it displays antigen fragments bound to its unique MHC molecules

This combination of antigen and MHC attracts the help of a mature matching T-cell.

Cytokines secreted by the T-cell help the B-cell to multiply and mature into antibody producing plasma cells.

Released into the blood, antibodies lock onto matching antigens. The antigen-antibody complexes are then cleared by the complement cascade or by the liver and spleen.

**Figure 2: B Cell Activation and Antibody Generation**

*Image credit: Fred the Oyster / Public domain*
*https://upload.wikimedia.org/wikipedia/commons/6/6a/B_cell_activation.svg*

---

[34] Gabrielli S, Ortolani C, del Zotto G, et al. The memories of NK cells: Innate-adaptive immune intrinsic crosstalk. *J Immuno Res*, 2016 Dec 19; http://dx.doi.org/10.1155/2016/1376595

[35] Netea MG, Latz E, et al. Innate immune memory: a paradigm shift in understanding host defense. *Nat Immunology*, 2015 Jul, 16(7): 675-679.

It must be kept in mind that there are many molecules involved in the immune response besides antibodies (including interferons, cytokines, chemokines, and even the antigens which are present on pathogens), many cellular responses besides antibody generation (including cell-to-cell initiation of programmed cell death, engulfing of pathogens or damaged cells, and regulation of other immune cells), and newly emerging roles attributed to the microbiome[36,37,38] and the virome[39] in immune health and function. In addition, nutrition plays a vital role in the maintenance of the immune system.[40] Thus, it is an inappropriate oversimplification to think that we can mimic the coordinated array of natural immune responses by targeting B cells and measuring the body's production of antibodies produced in response to a vaccine.

## Problems that Arise in Immune Function

The immune system is an amazingly coordinated array of cells, organs, and molecules, but it can malfunction. There are two types of malfunctions that are key to our understanding of the mechanism of vaccination and related concerns about vaccine safety. These are allergic reactions and autoimmune disorders.

### Allergic Reactions

An allergic reaction (or hypersensitivity response) occurs when a person is exposed to a harmless substance that the body "misidentifies" as a pathogen. The allergen then triggers a full-blown immune response, which is generally a result of the deployment of a specific type of antibody (IgE) against the allergen. It is sometimes possible to "outgrow" an allergy, but it is also possible that continual exposure to the allergen (and the accompanying inflammation of the tissues affected by the release of IgE and histamine, another molecule responsible for the effects of allergic reactions) can cause permanent damage and even lead to remodeling of body tissues that have a negative impact on the individual.[41]

The mechanism of allergies raises another important point that should be mentioned about the immune system – it is really the actions of the body itself in trying to destroy or expel a pathogen that gives us the feeling of "being sick," and not the direct action of the pathogen. Fevers, runny noses, body aches, coughing, and other symptoms are usually a direct result of the proper functioning of the immune system.[42] The exception to this rule is when the pathogen produces a

---

[36] Levy M, Kolodziejczyk AA, Thaiss CA, Elinav E. Dysbiosis and the immune system. *Nat Rev Immunol*, 2017; 17: 219–232. https://doi.org/10.1038/nri.2017.7

[37] Shi N, Li N, Duan X, et al. Interaction between the gut microbiome and mucosal immune system. *Military Med Res*, 2017; 4(14). https://doi.org/10.1186/s40779-017-0122-9

[38] Thaiss C, Zmora N, Levy M. et al. The microbiome and innate immunity. *Nature*, 2016; 535: 65–74. https://doi.org/10.1038/nature18847
A multitude of other papers on this subject could also be cited.

[39] Mukhopadhya I, Segal JP, Carding SR, et al. The gut virome: The 'missing link' between gut bacteria and host immunity? *Therapeutic Advances in Gastroenterology*, 2019 Mar 25; https://doi.org/10.1177/1756284819836620

[40] Marcos A, Nova E, Montero A. Changes in the immune system are conditioned by nutrition. *Eur J Clin Nutr*, 2003; 57: S66–S69. https://doi.org/10.1038/sj.ejcn.1601819
Again, many more papers could be cited on this subject.

[41] Murphy K, Travers P, Walport M. *Janeway's Immunobiology, 9th Ed*. New York and London: Garland Science, Taylor & Francis Group, 2017, p. 602-627.

[42] National Academy of Sciences. How Pathogens Make Us Sick. http://needtoknow.nas.edu/id/infection/how-pathogens-make-us-sick/ Accessed 18 May 2020.

toxin, like the tetanus toxin, that causes other painful (and potentially life-threatening) symptoms in the body. Nevertheless, the general rule holds true across a wide variety of both infectious and chronic diseases. Thus, one of the purported advantages of vaccines is that they bypass the full activation of the immune system, triggering immunological memory without the suffering inherent in actually contracting an illness. We will subsequently unpack the truth of both parts of this claim.

## Autoimmune Disorders

Autoimmune responses are mediated somewhat differently than hypersensitivity reactions, and can involve misdirected antibodies or problems with T cells. However, the underlying problem of reacting to a non-threatening substance is essentially the same. Autoimmunity can be broadly explained as a "misidentification" of the body's own tissues as pathogens. This is thought to involve a breakdown in the recognition of "self." Under normal conditions, the body has a mechanism for eliminating immune cells that are too "self-reactive" through screening and programmed cell death.* However, it is thought that sometimes cells that are autoreactive slip past all of the body's "checkpoints" and become activated. If this happens with a few cells, the body's normal mechanisms can handle the situation and all is happily resolved. Nevertheless, sometimes, for reasons that are still not entirely known, a sustained self-reaction results, and the immune system begins making many cells that attack and destroy tissues within the body.[43] This form of immune dysregulation is growing increasingly more common: autoimmune conditions are now the third leading cause of disease in the United States.[44]

Since vaccines seek to activate the immune system in novel ways that the body does not encounter under normal circumstances, it is important to investigate the potential role of vaccines in initiating both hypersensitivity responses and the autoimmune cascade. Both of these situations will be addressed in more detail in a later section. The next few sections of this chapter will address the three main biological issues that indicate that vaccine policy is increasingly out-of-step with our current understanding of the biology of the immune system.

## *Artificial Standards: Antibodies Do Not Equal Immunity*

In a sentence, it can be said that the overarching goal of vaccination is to bypass the body's natural immune mechanism (and all of its unpleasant and messy symptoms) and elicit a response within a

---

* In order to communicate with other immune cells, an individual immune cell must have some ability to recognize the markers on other cells, i.e. it must be somewhat self-reactive. But it cannot be *too* self-reactive, or it will begin to turn its lethal action (normally directed only against pathogens) on the body's own cells.

     The current understanding of how immune cells are produced suggests that the molecules involved in cell-to-cell recognition and in antibody production are formed through a process that involves randomized rearrangement of genetic material. This causes each immune cell to have unique properties and to be uniquely reactive to particular antigens. In the process of this random formation, about ¾ of the cells that are produced will react either too strongly or too weakly with the body's tissues and will be eliminated through the process of programmed cell death. As described, this genetic rearrangement would result in an almost limitless amount of variation among immune cells, and is designed to give man the ability to maximize his protection against pathogens.

[43] Murphy K, Travers P, Walport M. *Janeway's Immunobiology, 9th Ed.* New York and London: Garland Science, Taylor & Francis Group, 2017, p. 643-652.

[44] Cave S. *What Your Doctor May* Not *Tell You about Children's Vaccinations.* New York: Grand Central Publishing, 2010, p. 90-91.

15

specific facet of the final line of immunological defense, the B cells that produce antibodies. The opening article in *Plotkin's Vaccines*, the premier textbook on vaccination, states:

> Vaccine-induced immune effectors are essentially antibodies—produced by B lymphocytes—capable of binding specifically to a toxin or a pathogen.[45]

Vaccine effectiveness is measured by an antibody titer,* a test to determine just how much antibody to a specific pathogen is being produced in an individual. The absence of antibodies is often considered evidence that the individual is no longer immune to the disease, and generally leads to a recommendation for a re-inoculation (booster shot). But this marker alone may not be an accurate indication that real, long-lasting immunity to the pathogen has been obtained.

Dr. Tetyana Obukhanych makes a compelling case that our understanding of the nature of the immune system and its operations has been hampered by a focus on antibodies. She cites the early use of horse anti-serum as a treatment for diphtheria/tetanus as the origin of our belief in the antibody hypothesis. The horses were injected with increasing doses of the toxin, up to what would normally be a lethal dose, but they did not die because their bodies had been habituated to the toxin by the gradual increase in dosage. Instead, they produced an effective immune response; their serum was then collected and injected into humans to treat them for the same disease.[46] Similar experiments were conducted in other animal models: guinea pigs were protected against diphtheria toxin using anti-serum from recently vaccinated guinea pigs, and mice were protected against tetanus toxin using blood from tetanus-immune rabbits.[47] The anti-toxic effect of the serum was attributed to the presence of antibodies to the diphtheria and tetanus toxins.

Horse serum was not well-tolerated by humans and scientists soon discovered an alternative method for producing antibodies. This involved treating the toxins with formaldehyde (creating toxoids) and injecting them directly into human patients. The patients developed antibodies to the toxoids and early immunologic tests found that the two types of antibodies (those produced in the horse to the toxin and those produced in the humans to the toxoid) had similar reactivity to the toxin *in vitro* (that is, outside the body of the actual organism, and outside the context of the immune system as a whole).[48] Immunologists thus concluded that the immune responses elicited by the two procedures were equivalent, apparently without testing this theory *in vivo*.

Whenever a scientist wishes to establish that there is a causal connection between a variable and an outcome (in this case between the antibodies present in the serum and the patient's recovery

---

[45] Siegrist CA. Vaccine Immunology. In: Plotkin SA, Offit, PA, Orenstein WA, Edwards KM. *Plotkin's Vaccines, 7th ed.* Philadelphia: Elsevier, 2018, p. 16-34.

* The actual test is generally performed only when there is a question as to whether a person was vaccinated or whether they are still immune (for example, pregnant women might be tested for antibodies to rubella if they are concerned about congenital rubella syndrome). Tests are not conducted on a routine basis to determine the efficacy of vaccines after they are given by a pediatrician, nor to determine whether it is appropriate to continue to give boosters to children. (*see* Cave, Stephanie. *What Your Doctor May Not Tell You about Children's Vaccinations.* New York: Grand Central Publishing, 2010, p. 11-12)

[46] Obukhanych T. *Vaccine Illusion.* Amazon Digital Services LLC, 2012.

[47] Slifka MK and Amanna IJ. Passive Immunization. In: Plotkin SA, Offit, PA, Orenstein WA, Edwards KM. *Plotkin's Vaccines, 7th ed.* Philadelphia: Elsevier, 2018, p. 84-95.

[48] Obukhanych T. *Vaccine Illusion.* Amazon Digital Services LLC, 2012.

from tetanus or diphtheria), he must conduct a comparison of outcomes between two groups: one group who receives the variable (the antibody-containing horse serum) and one group who does not (in this case, a group who received everything in the horse serum except the antibody). Because of the serious side effects of the horse serum, the experiment just described would have been unethical and was never completed; but neither were analogous experiments that could have been done in animal models. As a consequence, the direct one-to-one link between antibodies and immunity was never fully established, but only assumed.[49] Please note: asserting that this link between antibodies and immunity is a foundational assumption does not constitute a denial that antibodies play a role in successful immune function, nor that antibodies may be used successfully for immunotherapy (under certain conditions).[50,51]

It is particularly important to note the two pathogens that were used in the original anti-sera experiments, diphtheria and tetanus, are not representative of the type of pathogens that are generally vaccinated against today. Both of these pathogens produce damaging toxins which can be bound by antibodies (specifically, by IgG and IgA)[52] and thus "neutralized," or prevented from damaging the tissue of the affected individual. This is not the case for all pathogens, and experiments using injected antibodies to create an immediate form of "passive" immunity to bacteria that are not toxin-producing have either varied efficacy or none at all.[53] These facts alone should cast considerable doubt on the antibody hypothesis, as it is clear that the antibodies to different kinds of pathogens produce different outcomes in the body. If a single type of pathogen was favored in the original experiments with horse serum, as we have seen, it could easily have given rise to a short-sighted fixation on a single molecule (antibodies) as a marker of total immunity.

Further evidence that immunologists might be on the wrong track about immunity being equivalent to antibody response comes from a number of case studies where two surprising outcomes were observed. In some cases, individuals with no antibody detectable in their system still showed no detectable antibody after receiving boosters, and even experienced severe reactions to re-vaccination that indicated their bodies were already sufficiently primed to the disease and their immunological memory was quite robust.[54] In other cases, individuals with detectable antibody not only contracted – but actually died – of the disease from which they were supposedly protected,[55] and mothers gave birth to babies with congenital rubella syndrome even though their antibody titers suggested they were immune to rubella.[56] Here we have strong *in vivo* evidence suggesting that antibodies alone are insufficient to establish or indicate the lasting resistance to a pathogen which is properly called immunity.

---

[49] Ibid.

[50] Slifka MK and Amanna IJ. Passive Immunization. In: Plotkin SA, Offit, PA, Orenstein WA, Edwards KM. *Plotkin's Vaccines, 7th ed.* Philadelphia: Elsevier, 2018, p. 84-95.

[51] Keller MA, Stiehm ER. Passive Immunity in Prevention and Treatment of Infectious Diseases. *Clin Micro Rev,* 2000 Oct; 13(4): 602-614. doi: 10.1128/CMR.13.4.602

[52] Murphy K, Travers P, Walport M. *Janeway's Immunobiology, 9th Ed.* New York and London: Garland Science, Taylor & Francis Group, 2017, p. 426-428.

[53] Keller MA, Stiehm ER. Passive Immunity in Prevention and Treatment of Infectious Diseases. *Clin Micro Rev,* 2000 Oct; 13(4): 602-614. doi: 10.1128/CMR.13.4.602

[54] Moskowitz R. *Vaccines: A Reappraisal.* New York: Skyhorse Publishing, 2017, p.24-27.

[55] Obukhanych T. *Vaccine Illusion.* Amazon Digital Services LLC, 2012.

[56] Diodati CJM. *Immunization: History, Ethics, Law and Health*, Ontario, CN: Integral Aspects Incorporated, 1999, p. 32

## Artificial Induction of the Immune System

In addition to the problematic lack of correlation between antibodies and immunity, the very idea that we can bypass the first defenses of the immune system and produce something akin to natural immunity by introducing a pathogen (or pathogen components) through injection is problematic.

The administration of vaccines is ultimately an artificial exposure to an antigen. This is, in part, because the injection of a vaccine intramuscularly* bypasses the normal routes of pathogen entry into the body, which causes immune responses to occur in different tissues than where they would occur in a normal infection. It has been known for at least two decades that immune cells in the muscle will not produce the same response as immune cells in the mucosal lining of the respiratory system and digestive tract.[57,58] One of the promising aspects of the technology that first interested me in vaccinations was a proposal to rectify this situation through the production of edible vaccines. These would have presented the antigen to the immune system through the oral route, which is a major route of infection for at least some pathogens. Though these vaccines never materialized, other vaccines have been developed that are administered directly to the mucosal system. These vaccines also demonstrate that vaccination in one area of the mucous membranes does not necessarily equate to an immune response in other areas of the body, or even other areas of the mucous membranes.[59] In fact, immune responses seem to be quite localized to particular areas after administration of mucosal vaccines,[60] and this remains an obstacle to their use; they simply do not give the same antibody titers as their intramuscular counterparts and are therefore judged to be deficient.

Other factors that contribute to the artificiality of vaccine-induced responses are two effects vaccines have on the cellular aspects of the immune system: they fail to activate the innate arm of the immune system and they tip the balance of immune activation heavily in favor of antibody-

---

* Two exceptions to the intramuscular route are the oral polio vaccine and the nasal influenza vaccine. Both vaccines have questionable efficacy – the oral polio vaccine is the source of more cases of polio-induced paralysis than wild polio virus, and the flu vaccine was pulled from the US market in 2016 because it provided roughly 3% protection against the flu virus. The vaccine was allowed to be administered in the US again in 2018, but is still highly ineffective. *For the oral polio vaccine, see:* https://www.the-scientist.com/news-opinion/polio-vaccination-causes-more-infections-than-wild-virus-66778
*See also:* https://apnews.com/7d8b0e32efd0480fbd12acf27729f6a5
*For the nasal flu vaccine, see:* https://www.nbcnews.com/health/health-news/flumist-nasal-flu-vaccine-can-come-back-vaccine-advisers-say-n849986

[57] Manrique M, Kozlowski P, Wang S, et al. Nasal DNA-MVA SIV vaccination provides more significant protection from progression to AIDS than a similar intramuscular vaccination. *Mucosal Immunol*, 2009; 2: 536–550. https://doi.org/10.1038/mi.2009.103

[58] Aase A, Naess LM, Sandin RH, et al. Comparison of functional immune responses in humans after intranasal and intramuscular immunisations with outer membrane vesicle vaccines against group B meningococcal disease. *Vaccine*, 2003 May 16; 21(17-18): 2042-2051.

     While this paper argues that the mucosal route does not demonstrate as robust an immune response as the intramuscular route, they are using only antibody titers to measure protection (which, as we have seen, may not be accurate measures). However, their findings still demonstrate the important point that there is a significant difference in the reaction of the immune system to different routes of challenge by vaccines.

[59] Kiyono H, Fukuyama S. NALT- versus Peyer's-patch-mediated mucosal immunity. *Nat Rev Immunol*. 2004; 4(9): 699–710. doi:10.1038/nri1439

[60] Holmgren, J., Czerkinsky, C. Mucosal immunity and vaccines. *Nat Med* (2005); 11: S45–S53. https://doi.org/10.1038/nm1213

producing B cells over other cells that are involved in cellular immunity. The latter point will be addressed first.

As repeatedly stated in *Plotkin's Vaccines*, antibodies are universally considered to be the effector mechanism of interest in vaccination. Despite its lack of rigorous experimental verification, the antibody hypothesis continues to drive the development of vaccines and the way that their efficacy is measured in clinical environments. This is particularly evident when one considers that of the 31 types of licensed vaccines, IgG antibodies are considered the primary correlates of immunity for 28 of the 31 types, with additional IgA antibodies correlating to three out of 28. In contrast, only four vaccines are definitely correlated with an increase in T cell activity as a marker of immune protection.[61] However, these correlates may or may not be related to protective immunity – either against infection by the pathogen or against the development of the disease after infection.[62] While in some instances it seems clear which effector molecules result in protection after vaccination, in other instances it is assumed because the actual mechanism is difficult to prove.[63] The bias towards studying antibody responses may, in fact, be preventing the discovery of alternative effector mechanisms – and it is possible that the process of artificially exposing organisms to injected pathogens during immunological studies has actually given us an incorrect understanding of immune responses altogether. What we have observed in the laboratory has been artificial immune responses, not natural ones.[64] It is also possible that the amount of antibodies produced in response to vaccination is in excess of what the body would normally require to effectively clear a pathogen, and this would likely mediate other types of pathology (which will be discussed in more detail in the section on vaccine safety).

In addition, certain types of vaccines that do not persist for long periods in the body are unlikely to generate efficient memory responses in T cells due to the short duration of exposure to the antigen.[65] This may also result in poorer quality memory T cells, which are not as effective in responding to infection.[66] As cell-mediated immunity (both through T cells and through NK cells) is an important part of clearing infections in the body, tipping the scales of the adaptive immune system away from cellular immunity can lead to a reduction in the immune system's capacity to handle infection once a pathogen has taken hold. This means that if a vaccine fails to prevent infection, it may actually hinder recovery from a disease.

Contributing additionally to this artificiality is the fact that by activating the adaptive immune system without the innate immune system, vaccination actually works in reverse order of the body's design. It is possible that this may cause an overall atrophy of the innate immune response, as it is no longer "primed" by normal exposure to childhood infectious agents.[67] If this occurs, it would further diminish the body's ability to respond to any pathogens it is not vaccinated against.

---

[61] Siegrist CA. Vaccine Immunology. In: Plotkin SA, Offit, PA, Orenstein WA, Edwards KM. *Plotkin's Vaccines, 7th ed.* Philadelphia: Elsevier, 2018, p. 16-34.

[62] Plotkin SA and Gilbert P. Corrrelates of Protection. In: Plotkin SA, Offit, PA, Orenstein WA, Edwards KM. *Plotkin's Vaccines, 7th ed.* Philadelphia: Elsevier, 2018, p. 35-40.

[63] Ibid.

[64] *See:* Obukhanych T. *Vaccine Illusion.* Amazon Digital Services LLC, 2012

[65] Siegrist CA. Vaccine Immunology. In: Plotkin SA, Offit, PA, Orenstein WA, Edwards KM. *Plotkin's Vaccines, 7th ed.* Philadelphia: Elsevier, 2018, p. 16-34.

[66] Ibid.

[67] Moskowitz R. *Vaccines: A Reappraisal.* New York: Skyhorse Publishing, 2017, p. 16.

This could explain the findings of some physicians that children who are "under-vaccinated" tend to have fewer emergency room visits for acute illness, as well as fewer outpatient visits to physicians, particularly for respiratory infections.[68] If vaccines are suppressing immune response to non-vaccinated illness, this is the trend we would expect to see.

There is one final problem with artificially activating the immune system that is often overlooked. Stimulating immune responses to specific pathogens may "over-commit" our immune resources in the direction of a particular set of diseases, and this may leave us more vulnerable overall to other diseases for which we are not being vaccinated.[*] In general, it is important to remember that though the hyper-variable genetics of the immune cells give the body's immune system what appears to be a limitless capacity to recognize and remember different types of pathogens, the resources of the immune system are finite. Our bodies are finite, and to the extent that time, energy, and material resources are committed to one activity, they are withdrawn from another. You have experienced this every time you have eaten a large meal – the resultant sleepiness you feel after Thanksgiving dinner is not due to the tryptophan in the turkey, but due to the re-allocation of blood flow and other resources to the digestive system, which now has a great deal of work to do to break down the day's dainties. Analogously, if the immune system is primed to commit to engaging with specific pathogens in a certain way, resources are not available for other pathogens.

### The Changing Understanding of the Human Immune System Compounds the Problem of Artificially Induced Immunity

The focus of vaccine development and efficacy studies up to this point has remained on the antibody hypothesis in part because B cells (which produce antibodies) are a part of the adaptive immune system and thought to be a primary cell type involved with immunological memory. Many studies have been done, both *in vitro* and *in vivo*, examining the nature of memory B cells and memory T cells.[69] Recent evidence has provided a reason to shift our thinking about the cellular components of immunological memory, however, and to include natural killer (NK) cells and monocytes (two major types of innate immune cells) as important players in immunological memory.[70]

As mentioned, innate immune cells were initially considered irrelevant to the body's immunological memory. Recent research has suggested that this view is incorrect and that these cells are actively protecting against reinfection by previously encountered pathogens.[71] This

---

[68] Glanz JM, Newcome SR, et al. A population-based cohort study of undervaccination in 8 managed care organizations across the United States. *JAMA Pediatr* 2013 Mar 1; 167(3): 274-81.

[*] There are numerous examples of this phenomenon that will be discussed in the following pages: vaccination against pertussis leaves us vulnerable to parapertussis, vaccination against chickenpox leaves us vulnerable to shingles, and vaccination against the wrong strain of seasonal influenza leaves us vulnerable to other strains.

[69] Murphy K, Travers P, Walport M. *Janeway's Immunobiology, 9th Ed*. New York and London: Garland Science, Taylor & Francis Group, 2017, p. 473-485.

[70] Netea MG, Joosten LAB, Latz E, et al. Trained immunity: a program of innate immune memory in health and disease. *Science*. 2016 April 22; 352(6284): aaf1098. doi:10.1126/science.aaf1098.

[71] Netea MG, Joosten LAB, et al. Trained immunity: a program of innate immune memory in health and disease. *Science* 2016 April 22; 352(6284): doi:10.1126/science.aaf1098.

process is mediated by epigenetic* changes in the immune cells, and may even take place in progenitor cells (cells that are very early in their development and have not yet differentiated into their final form). Our understanding of epigenetics is changing as quickly or more quickly than our understanding of the immune system, and this adds an additional layer of complexity for understanding the process of acquiring immunity. Protection against reinfection has also been observed in organisms that lack adaptive cells entirely, lending additional support to the idea that immunity is mediated by more than just antibody response or T cell activation.[72]

There is also a tremendous body of new evidence suggesting an important role for the microbiome** in the complex function of the immune system. Researchers are still unsure exactly what constitutes "healthy" gut flora, as the makeup of a microbiome in an individual who is free from disease can vary according to geographic region, diet, method of colonization, and other factors.[73] It may seem self-evident that the immune system would regulate the bacteria, viruses, fungi, and protists that colonize the human body, but the microbes also regulate the immune system in a continual feedback loop. This can have profound impacts on health, as imbalances in the gut bacteria that are associated with disease states can become self-maintaining by modulating the immune response to favor the growth of harmful microbes.[74] Much of the feedback that occurs between the immune system and the microbiome is mediated by antibodies (specifically IgA) and this raises an additional area of concern. If current vaccines are manipulating the antibody response as their primary target, we do not know what profound effects this may have on the microbiome.

*Not All Vaccinations Are Equal*

An additional source of confusion about vaccination is that there are several different methods of producing the active ingredients in a vaccine, and these different methods all have different risks and counter-indications. It will be helpful before we continue our discussion to briefly explain the three main types of vaccine preparations, which are *live-attenuated*, *inactivated*, and *subunit*

---

* A relatively new field in biology (it began gaining significant ground in research in the 1990s), epigenetics is a study of the complex interaction between genes and their environments (both locally within the cell, and exterior to the organism as a whole). Prior to the recent research into epigenetics, scientists mainly thought that the sequence of genes dictated our anatomy and physiology. We now know that the physical structure of the genes can be modified at a number of different levels, resulting in differing expression of the gene (which then has a profound impact on the organism whose genes are so altered). Exactly how this works is still incompletely understood.

[72] Ibid.

** While some websites incorrectly assert that bacteria cells outnumber human cells in the body by 10:1, it is true that we are probably outnumbered. More accurate estimates give a roughly 1.3:1 ratio, though even this is still being debated. (See: "Revised Estimates for the Number of Human and Bacterial Cells in the Body", https://journals.plos.org/plosbiology/article?id=10.1371/journal.pbio.1002533) The collection of all the bacterial cells that live in and on our bodies is referred to as the "microbiome," and it has been implicated in everything from gut health to emotional disorders. Much research remains to be done to pin down all of the effects of the interactions between our bodies and our microbiomes.

[73] Levy M, Kolodziejczyk AA, Thaiss CA, Elinav E. Dysbiosis and the immune system. *Nat Rev Immunol*, 2017; 17: 219–232. https://doi.org/10.1038/nri.2017.7

[74] Levy M, Kolodziejczyk AA, Thaiss CA, Elinav E. Dysbiosis and the immune system. *Nat Rev Immunol*, 2017; 17: 219–232. https://doi.org/10.1038/nri.2017.7

vaccines.[75]  The latter group includes a specific subset called *toxoid* vaccines that deserve additional explanation as they have some unique properties.

Live-attenuated vaccines are a weakened form of a regular pathogen and consist of whole cells or virus particles.  As such, they are capable of continuing to replicate in the human body once the vaccine has been delivered.  This is thought to boost their ability to elicit a protective immune response, as they are able to persist in the body for a longer period of time than other vaccines.[76]  It can also lead to a problem peculiar to live vaccines called *shedding*, which occurs when recipients of the vaccine actually pass live, active pathogens into the environment.[77, 78]  It is possible to contract infection from the live viruses that are shed, and so vaccinated persons can pass a disease on to susceptible individuals (particularly to infants and those with compromised immune systems) for several weeks to several months after receiving a vaccination.[79]  It is also possible for the vaccinated person himself to contract the disease* from the vaccine.[80]

Inactivated vaccines (sometimes also referred to as "killed" vaccines) contain the whole pathogen, but in an inactive form.  This inactivation is usually accomplished by the addition of chemicals such as formaldehyde.[81]  One advantage of this form of vaccine is that the shedding process described above does not occur; a disadvantage is that the active component of the vaccine does not persist as long in the body and so does not elicit as strong of an antibody response.[82]  This lowered response can result in vaccine failure, a process that will be discussed in more detail in a subsequent section.  Another serious disadvantage of this method is that some pathogens are resistant to formaldehyde inactivation, and can escape live and intact.[83]  In this case, the vaccine could also give the vaccinated person the disease, but this is more likely to be batch-specific than vaccine-specific.

Subunit vaccines use pieces of the pathogen as "markers" to elicit an immune response.  It is thought that these specific markers (antigens), give the immune system a sufficient signal to later recognize the whole infectious agent.  Usually these antigens are proteins or complex sugars.  The toxoid vaccines are a special category of subunit vaccines that use molecules that the pathogens produce and secrete rather than molecules that make up the cell of the actual pathogens themselves.  This, in theory, should cause the body to mount an immune response against the toxin, which would be helpful in controlling the side-effects of an infection, but may prove ineffective against

---

[75] U.S. Department of Health and Human Services. "Vaccine Types," https://www.vaccines.gov/basics/types Accessed 17 Aug 2019

[76] World Health Organization, "Vaccine Safety Basics," https://vaccine-safety-training.org/live-attenuated-vaccines.html Accessed 24 Aug 2019.

[77] Moskowitz R. *Vaccines: A Reappraisal*. New York: Skyhorse Publishing, 2017, p. 23.

[78] Miller NZ. *Miller's Review of Critical Vaccine Studies*. Santa Fe: New Atlantean Press, 2016, p 143.

[79] Humphries S and Bystrianyk R. *Dissolving Illusions*. Printed by author. 2015, p 347-356.

* "Atypical measles" is one example.  Infection by polio from the oral polio vaccine is another.

[80] Ibid, p 347-356.

[81] Centers for Disease Control and Prevention. "What's in Vaccines?" https://www.cdc.gov/vaccines/vac-gen/additives.htm Accessed 24 Aug 2019.

Ingredients for US licensed vaccines can be found on the package inserts, and are also compiled at this website: https://vaccines.procon.org/vaccine-ingredients-and-manufacturer-information/

[82] U.S. Department of Health and Human Services. "Vaccine Types," https://www.vaccines.gov/basics/types Accessed 17 Aug 2019.

[83] Humphries S and Bystrianyk R. *Dissolving Illusions*. Printed by author. 2015, p 272-276.

clearing the actual pathogen from the body. The primary advantage of subunit vaccines is that there is no way to contract the actual disease; the primary disadvantage is that the material is cleared from the body even more quickly than the inactivated vaccines, and produces the weakest immune response of the three types. This generally leads to the necessity for more doses of the vaccine.[84] These vaccines also contain materials known as *adjuvants*, which are molecules that are designed to heighten the immune response to the vaccine antigen. When concerns are expressed about the safety of vaccine ingredients, they often involve questions about the adjuvants.

| Live-Attenuated Vaccines | Inactivated Vaccines | Subunit Vaccines |
|---|---|---|
| Measles | Hepatitis A | Hib (Haemophilus influenzae type b) |
| Mumps | Influenza (intramuscular) | Hepatitis B |
| Rubella | Polio (injected) | HPV |
| Rotavirus | Rabies | Pertussis (DTaP vaccine) |
| Chickenpox | Typhoid | Pneumococcal disease |
| Smallpox | Cholera | Meningococcal disease |
| Yellow fever | | Shingles |
| Polio (oral) | | Tetanus (toxoid) |
| Influenza (nasal) | | Diphtheria (toxoid) |
| BCG (tuberculosis) | | |

**Table 1:  Vaccines by Type[85]**

## Vaccination and Immunity are Not Equivalent

The layers of complexity just described concerning innate immunity, epigenetics, and the microbiome exponentially compound the problem of understanding how to safely and effectively initiate artificially-acquired immunity. The complexity even calls into question whether the response induced by artificial means can appropriately be called "immunity." In order to have complete, lasting immunity, it is becoming increasingly apparent that the whole immune system needs to be involved in the process of building immunological memory. Vaccination, which focuses on the antibody response and comes with a variety of disadvantages associated with each method of producing a vaccine, is clearly an insufficient mechanism to produce real immunity to a pathogen.

---

[84] U.S. Department of Heatlh and Human Services. "Vaccine Types," https://www.vaccines.gov/basics/types , accessed 17 Aug 2019
[85] Data taken from:  U.S. Department of Heatlh and Human Services. "Vaccine Types," https://www.vaccines.gov/basics/types Accessed 17 Aug 2019. and Cave S. *What Your Doctor May* Not *Tell You about Children's Vaccinations*. New York: Grand Central Publishing, 2010, p. 9-10.

# The Limitations of Vaccination

*Oddly enough, it appears that the only reason to continue mass immunization*
*against poliomyelitis is to try to make up for the loss of passive immunity*
*resulting from decades of vaccine use.*
*-- Catherine J. M. Diodati, MA*[86]

In addition to the mechanisms of natural immunity being poorly understood (and therefore very difficult to manipulate predictably using artificial methods), there are other biological limitations to vaccination. Despite assertions in popular media, vaccination as a method of inducing acquired immunity is neither permanent nor failsafe. This chapter will address the limitations of vaccines on three fronts: the transitory nature of the artificial immunity conferred by vaccines, the fact that vaccines fail to confer immunity at all in certain cases, and the need for additional chemicals called adjuvants in order to make some vaccines elicit any response from the immune system.

## *The Induction of Immunity by Vaccination Is Temporary*

The most popular myth circulated involving immunological memory is the idea that the immune response produced by vaccines is life-long, or (failing that) is at least as long-lasting as an immune response induced by exposure to an actual disease.[87] This is partly due to a mistaken understanding of the nature of vaccination as somehow truly mimicking natural infection. Yet, as we saw in the previous section, this is manifestly not the case. We now know that even natural immunity does not always last forever, but we have long known that vaccinations are much more short-lived in terms of protectiveness than a natural infection. Physicians in Jenner's day recognized that ongoing "boosters" were required to maintain vaccine-induced protection against infection, and that permanent immunity was never reached through vaccination. Some striking modern examples of this lack of permanence include the following:

> A study found that 38% of recipients of a Hepatitis B vaccine showed extremely low antibody levels just three years after their initial vaccination.[88]

> At least 35% of the recipients of the HPV vaccine had undetectable antibodies after 5 years.[89] Given that most girls are vaccinated beginning at age 11, this potentially means that up to 1/3 of the women who receive the vaccine will have lost immunity prior to becoming at risk for contracting the disease.

> The World Health Organization reported that "25% to 60% of adults will lose all detectable antibody to hepatitis B vaccine within 6 to 10 years." Though there was not data available for children at the time that this fact was reported, it is not unreasonable to conclude that

---

[86] Diodati CJM. *Immunization: History, Ethics, Law and Health.* Ontario, CN: Integral Aspects Incorporated, 1999, p. 131.

[87] Murphy K, Travers P, and Walport M. *Janeway's Immunobiology, 9th Ed.* New York and London: Garland Science, Taylor & Francis Group, 2017, p. 472-474.

[88] Horowitz MM, Ershler WB, McKinney WP, et al. Duration of Immunity After Hepatitis B Vaccination: Efficacy of Low-Dose Booster Vaccine. *Ann Intern Med.* 1988; 108: 185–189. doi: 10.7326/0003-4819-108-2-185

[89] Vernon LF. How Silencing of Dissent in Science Impacts Woman. The Gardasil® Story. *Advances in Sexual Medicine,* 2017; 7: 179-204. *See also:* references 103 and 104 from the same paper.

the majority of infants who are now vaccinated for hepatitis B will have lost all antibody response by the time they are old enough to be at risk of contracting the disease.[90]

The Immunisation Advisory Centre of New Zealand has stated that diphtheria vaccines last approximately 10 years and pertussis** vaccines last only 4-6 years. Tetanus* vaccines may last up to 25 years, but at least a quarter of these vaccines only last 13-14 years.[91]

Most other vaccines for which we have data have only been tested up to 10-20 years after vaccination.[92] While it is possible that immunity is conferred on individuals past the 20-year mark, there is currently no evidence to support this claim. However, the careful reader may be asking themselves why, having just finished a long explanation of the many reasons that antibodies cannot by themselves stand as markers of immunity, there are now multiple statistics concerning antibodies offered to make a case against the lasting effectiveness of vaccines. These statistics show that even by vaccine proponents' own standards, vaccines fail to provide lasting immune protection.

Vaccine efficacy can also be examined by looking for evidence of disease outbreaks in highly vaccinated populations, which is a well-documented phenomenon. [93, 94, 95, 96, 97] In fact, for some diseases like measles, outbreaks in vaccinated populations[98] suggest that the loss of immunity in

---

[90] Diodati CJM. *Immunization: History, Ethics, Law and Health*. Ontario, CN: Integral Aspects Incorporated, 1999, p. 125.

** While pertussis immunity wanes even after natural infection (lasting only up to 20 years), the vaccine is clearly less effective than natural infection at producing lasting immunity, and could result in a child being re-infected with whooping cough while still at a relatively young age. (See Wendelboe AM, Van Rie A, Salmaso S, Englund JA. Duration of Immunity Against Pertussis After Natural Infection or Vaccination. *The Pediatric Infectious Disease Journal*: 2005 May; 24(5): S58-S61 doi: 10.1097/01.inf.0000160914.59160.41)

* While tetanus does not normally result in immunity through natural routes of infection (i.e. intramuscularly), studies from the 1920s showed that animals can attain immunity through exposure to tetanus spores in their guts. (See Obukhanych, 2012)

[91] The Immunisation Advisory Centre. "Efficacy and Effectiveness." Updated Jan 2020. https://www.immune.org.nz/vaccines/efficiency-effectiveness Accessed 18 April 2020.

[92] Ibid.

[93] Edmonson MB, Addiss DG, McPherson JT, Berg JL, Circo SR, Davis JP. Department of Pediatrics, University of Wisconsin, Madison 53792. Mild measles and secondary vaccine failure during a sustained outbreak in a highly vaccinated population. *JAMA*. 1990 May 9; 263(18): 2467-71.

[94] Vandermeulen C, Roelants M, Vermoere M, Roseeuw K, Goubau P, Hoppenbrouwers K. Department of Youth Health Care, Katholieke Universiteit Leuven, Kapucijnenvoer 35/1, 3000, Belgium. Outbreak Of Mumps In A Vaccinated Child Population: A Question Of Vaccine Failure? *Vaccine*. 2004 Jul 29; 22(21-22): 2713-6.

[95] Paunio M, Hedman K, Davidkin I, Valle M, Heinonen OP, Leinikki P, Salmi A, Peltola H. Department of Public Health, University of Helsinki, Finland. Secondary measles vaccine failures identified by measurement of IgG avidity: high occurrence among teenagers vaccinated at a young age. *Epidemiol Infect* 2000 Apr; 124(2): 263-71

[96] Briss PA, Fehrs LJ, Parker RA, Wright PF, Sannella EC, Hutcheson RH, and Schaffner W. Sustained Transmission of Mumps in a Highly Vaccinated Population: Assessment of Primary Vaccine Failure and Waning Vaccine-Induced Immunity, *J Infect Dis*, 1994 Jan; 169(1): 77–82, https://doi.org/10.1093/infdis/169.1.77

[97] A.V. Atrasheuskaya, M.V. Kulak, A.A. Neverov, S. Rubin, G.M. Ignatyev. [bMeasles Cases In Highly Vaccinated Population Of Novosibirsk, Russia, 2000-2005. *Vaccine*, 2008 Apr; 26(17) :2111-2118.

Many more articles could be cited here, and a search for "vaccine failure" on scholar.google.com (Oct 11, 2019) yielded more than 1.8 million hits.

[98] Rosen JB, Rota JS, et al. Outbreak of measles among persons with prior evidence of immunity, New York City, 2011. *Clin Infect Dis* 2014 May; 58(9): 1205-10

individuals (either before or after 20 years post-vaccination) is significant enough that diseases will continue to circulate in the population even when vaccination rates are very high. A few brief examples of such disease outbreaks in vaccinated populations are outlined below:

> While vaccine coverage levels have remained unchanged, both the UK and US have experienced a dramatic spike in the incidence of whooping cough since transitioning from the whole-cell pertussis vaccine to the acellular vaccine in the 1990s. The authors of the research on this subject even explicitly state: "It is clear that *waning immunity* plays a role in the epidemiology of *B. pertussis*, though estimates of the duration of protection to *B. pertussis* are highly varied."[99] [Emphasis added]

> Despite reporting 97.52% vaccination coverage achieved in 2010 (vaccination which was enforced regardless of immune status), China experienced 42,569 cases of measles in hundreds of separate outbreaks from 2011-2013. These cases were over 98% laboratory confirmed in 2012 and 2013, with percentages almost as high in 2011.[100]

> Mumps outbreaks have been rampant in the US in the last decade.[101] 2013 saw outbreaks of mumps on three different campuses in three different states: University of Richmond, Loyola University, and Fordham University. Reports indicated that these occurred in fully vaccinated (up to 100%) populations.[102] 484 cases of mumps were reported in central Ohio in 2014; this was the highest incidence of mumps cases in the region since 1979.[103] The University of Iowa and its surrounding communities reported 226 cases prior to an MMR vaccination campaign in 2015, and 75 cases after the campaign in 2016, despite a 98% vaccination rate (including 12% who had received a third dose of the MMR).[104] In 2016, a mumps outbreak at Harvard University involved at least 66 confirmed cases of mumps among students who were 98-99% vaccinated.[105] Massachusetts as a whole had over 250

---

[99] Althouse BM, Scarpino SV. Asymptomatic transmission and the resurgence of *Bordetella pertussis*. *BMC Med.* 2015; 13: 146. doi: 10.1186/s12916-015-0382-8

[100] Ma C, Hao L, Zhang Y, et al. Monitoring progress towards the elimination of measles in China: an analysis of measles surveillance data. *Bull World Health Organ*, 2014 May 1; 92(5): 340–347. doi: 10.2471/BLT.13.130195

[101] Wikipedia, while not a reliable news source generally, is certainly not a proponent of disseminating any information that could be used to discredit vaccines. Yet, they report at least 39 outbreaks of mumps in the US alone from 2005-2020, as well as other mumps outbreaks around the world.
See: https://en.wikipedia.org/wiki/Mumps_outbreaks_in_the_21st_century Accessed 11 May 2020.
See also: https://www.cdc.gov/mumps/outbreaks.html Accessed 11 May 2020.

[102] Bolinger T. *The Truth about Vaccines 2020: Episode 3*. TTAC.
https://go2.thetruthaboutvaccines.com/docuseries/replay/?utm_campaign=ttav&utm_medium=email&utm_source=all-actives-ttac&utm_content=replay-ttav-2020-may2-444pm&a_aid=5903de82cac79 Accessed 25 April 2020.

[103] City of Columbus. Mumps outbreak declared over in central Ohio – 10.10.2014. Columbus Public Health Press Release. 10 Oct 2014. < https://www.columbus.gov/publichealth/press/2014/Mumps-Outbreak-Declared-Over-in-Central-Ohio----10-10-2014/> Accessed 11 May 2020.

[104] Shah M, Quinlisk P, Weigel A, et al. Mumps Outbreak in a Highly Vaccinated University-Affiliated Setting Before and After a Measles-Mumps-Rubella Vaccination Campaign—Iowa, July 2015–May 2016. *Clin Infect Dis*, 2018 Jan 1: 66(1), 81–88. https://doi.org/10.1093/cid/cix718

[105] Narayanan MV and Shimozaki KK. Months After First Outbreak, Campus Rid of Mumps. *The Harvard Crimson*. 1 Sept 2016. < https://www.thecrimson.com/article/2016/9/1/mumps-gone-not-forgotten/> Accessed 11 May 2020.

cases of mumps in 2016 and over 170 cases in 2017.[106] The largest outbreaks in the decade were close to 3,000 people each: the first in 2009-2010 in New York City, and the second in 2016 in a small community in Arkansas.[107]

The cases just cited represent only the tip of the iceberg of disease outbreaks in highly vaccinated populations. For additional information, the reader can reference Dr. Richard Moskowitz's *Vaccines: A Reappraisal*, Dr. Suzanne Humphries' *Dissolving Illusions*, or almost any work by Neil Z. Miller.

## *The Induction of Immunity by Vaccination Is Ineffective: Vaccine Failure*

Outbreaks of disease in fully vaccinated populations may have an additional explanation besides a waning of vaccine-induced immunity. Research has revealed that a minimum of 2-10% of all vaccinated individuals fail to mount an antibody response to their initial vaccination.[108] This has been termed *primary vaccine failure*, and can be due to problems in vaccine manufacture or administration, or can be caused by a lack of receptivity due to the genetics or environment of the host. The situation discussed in the previous section, when individuals fail to maintain stable antibody titers, is termed *secondary vaccine failure*.

Both primary and secondary vaccine failure synergistically affect the ability of the population to attain a condition known as *herd immunity*. This is an ideal state in which a sufficient number of individuals are immune to a given disease, such that the disease no longer freely circulates in the population.[109] The more infectious a disease is, the higher the threshold of herd immunity is. For example, since measles can be spread through the air (making it much more contagious than something that has to be spread through bodily fluids or skin-to-skin contact), approximately 95% of individuals in a given population need to be immune to measles for the population as a whole to be able to contain a measles outbreak through herd immunity alone.[110, 111] However, the efficacy of the measles vaccine is estimated to be 85-99% after vaccine failure;[112] therefore, even with 100% vaccination coverage, it is probable that herd immunity might never be reached.•

---

[106] Zusl K. New details about mumps outbreaks of 2016-2017. *The Harvard Gazette*. 11 Feb 2020. < https://news.harvard.edu/gazette/story/2020/02/the-story-behind-the-mumps-outbreaks-of-2016-17/> Accessed 11 May 2020.

[107] CDC. Mumps cases and outbreaks. 11 Feb 2020. < https://www.cdc.gov/mumps/outbreaks.html> Accessed 11 May 2020.

[108] Wiedermann, U, Garner-Spitzer E, and A Wagner. Primary vaccine failure to routine vaccines: Why and what to do? *Hum Vaccin Immunother*. 2016 Jan; 12(1): 239–243.

[109] Helft L and Willingham E. "What is Herd Immunity?" NOVA. 5 Sept 2014. https://www.pbs.org/wgbh/nova/article/herd-immunity/ Accessed 18 Oct 2019.

[110] Ibid.

[111] Holland M, Zachary CE. Herd Immunity and Compulsory Childhood Vaccination: Does the Theory Justify the Law? *Oregon Law Review*, 2014; 93(1): 17.

[112] Holland M, Zachary CE. Herd Immunity and Compulsory Childhood Vaccination: Does the Theory Justify the Law? *Oregon Law Review*, 2014; 93(1): 17. (85-95%)

• Government of Canada. "Measles Vaccine: Canadian Immunization Guide," https://www.canada.ca/en/public-health/services/publications/healthy-living/canadian-immunization-guide-part-4-active-vaccines/page-12-measles-vaccine.html#p4c11a4 (Accessed 28 Oct 2019) suggests that booster doses may reach 100% efficacy, but this is unlikely given the average rate of vaccine failure and the poorly understood mechanisms of host incompatibility that contribute to failure rates. The article itself admits that measles outbreaks can and do occur in highly vaccinated populations, a fact that is consistent with at least some vaccine failure. This is particularly likely as these outbreaks

Another problem with vaccine failure that is generally not addressed occurs each year with the seasonal influenza (flu) vaccine. Since the vaccine cannot protect against all possible strains of the flu, vaccine developers must choose which strains they will incorporate into the vaccine each year based on patterns of strain circulation in the past. This guesswork means that in the best case scenario, the vaccine will fail 40-60% of the time, and in the worst case scenario the flu vaccine may fail to protect against the flu in up to 75-97% of cases. [113] In addition to this, the improper priming of the immune system with the wrong strains of the virus may actually make it more likely for a vaccinated individual to have worse clinical symptoms if they contract seasonal flu.[114, 115, 116, 117]

## *The Induction of Immunity by Vaccination Is Ineffective: The Need for Adjuvants*

The concept of subunit vaccines was previously introduced. While these vaccines are considered "safer" than both live and inactivated vaccines because they do not contain actual pathogens, this actually makes them much less effective than inactivated vaccines at producing an immune response. This is one of the reasons for the resurgence of whooping cough that was noted earlier.

To counter this disadvantage, subunit vaccines often include a component known as an *adjuvant* – a substance that heightens the body's immune response to a foreign antigen. Though their exact mechanism is not well understood, adjuvants may work in the body to activate certain proteins involved in immunity, recruit immune cells, or assist the immune cells to take up the active vaccine components.[118] Most vaccines that require adjuvants contain aluminum in one of the following forms: amorphous aluminum hydroxyphosphate sulfate (AAHS), aluminum hydroxide, aluminum phosphate, or potassium aluminum sulfate.[119]

Since 1911, the dangers of aluminum additives to foods (particularly baking soda) have been a subject of public discussion.[120] Given that oral absorption of aluminum is significantly lower than absorption from aluminum injected directly into the bloodstream, it is truly not a novel idea to

---

often occur in schools, where it is unlikely that any artificially-acquired immunity would already have waned (i.e. secondary vaccine failure is an unlikely culprit).

[113] Bloomberg. Why Flu Outbreaks Have Been the Worst in Nearly a Decade. *Time*, 28 Feb 2018. https://time.com/5179131/the-flu-vaccine-worst-year/ Accessed 21 April 2020.

[114] J.H. Kim, W.G. Davis, S. Sambhara and J. Jacob. Strategies to alleviate original antigenic sin responses to influenza viruses. PNAS (2012). doi: 10.1073/pnas.0912458109

[115] Kim JHK, Skoutzou I, Compans R, Jacob J. Original Antigenic Sin Response to Influenza Viruses. *J Immunol*, 2009; 183: 3294-3301. doi:10.4049/jimmunol.org/content/183/5/3294

[116] Khurana S, Loving CL, Manischewitz J, et al. Vaccine-Induced Anti-HA2 Antibodies Promote Virus Fusion and Enhance Influenza Virus Respiratory Disease. *Sci Translational Med,* 2013; 5(200). DOI: 10.1126/scitranslmed.3006366.

[117] Skowronski DN, De Serres G, Crowcroft NS, et al. Association between the 2008–09 Seasonal Influenza Vaccine and Pandemic H1N1 Illness during Spring–Summer 2009: Four Observational Studies from Canada. *PLOS Med,* 2010 Apr 6: https://doi.org/10.1371/journal.pmed.1000258.

[118] Awate S, Babiuk LA, and Mutwiri1G. Mechanisms of Action of Adjuvants. *Front Immunol.* 2013 May 16; 4: 114. doi: 10.3389/fimmu.2013.00114

[119] Centers for Disease Control and Prevention. "Adjuvants Help Vaccines Work Better." https://www.cdc.gov/vaccinesafety/concerns/adjuvants.html Accessed 19 Oct 2019.

[120] Shaw CA, Tomljenovic L. Aluminum in the central nervous system (CNS): toxicity in humans and animals, vaccine adjuvants, and autoimmunity. *Immunol Res* 2013 Jul: 56(2-3): 304-16.

suggest that aluminum adjuvants may be worrisome. The CDC claims that vaccine adjuvants have been used safely for decades, but ongoing research suggests that these aluminum-containing compounds are unsafe in the dosages that are given during the process of vaccination, and may have disproportionate negative impacts on populations that are susceptible to autoimmune disease.[121]

The FDA has published regulations regarding the administration of parenteral⁺ aluminum that indicate that the level of aluminum in vaccines is likely to be unsafe:

> Research indicates that patients with impaired kidney function, including premature neonates, who receive parenteral levels of aluminum at greater than 4 to 5 µg/kg/day accumulate aluminum at levels associated with central nervous system and bone toxicity. Tissue loading may occur at even lower rates of administration.[122]

This information is disconcerting because infants receive about 4.4 g of aluminum through vaccine adjuvants when the CDC vaccine schedule is followed from birth to six months.[123] While this may not seem like very much aluminum, it works out to about 24 µg/day, or 3.1 µg/kg/day for an average sized six month old, and 7.4 µg/kg/day for an average newborn. At first glance, this may not seem particularly alarming, as the dose for newborns is only slightly higher than the recommended safe dosage quoted in the passage above. However, these calculations do not tell the whole story; the aluminum is not injected in small doses over the course of the whole six months, but is injected all at once. Thus, the aluminum more readily accumulates in tissues because the body cannot effectively process that much aluminum at one time.

At birth, if an infant receives the hepatitis B vaccine, 250 µg of aluminum are administered into his body – in an average infant of about 3.4 kg[124], this would be 15-18 times the safe dose recommended by the FDA for that day's exposure. At two months, an average infant of about 5.5 kg will receive 1225 µg of aluminum in one day – this is 45-56 times the safe daily exposure rate from the FDA. Even allowing for the fact that the above recommendations are made for those who have kidney trouble, doses in these excessive ranges cannot be good for the body.

The doses of aluminum are especially troubling when one considers that aluminum from parenteral sources is unlikely to be cleared from the soft tissue (including the brain) in less than 100 days, and persists in bone tissue even longer [125] – and this data was obtained in adults, who are able to

---

[121] Moskowitz, Richard MD. *Vaccines: A Reappraisal.* New York: Skyhorse Publishing, 2017, p.76.
⁺ Parenteral is a medical term that means anything administered through a non-oral route.
[122] Electronic Code of Federal Regulations, Title 21, Section 201.323. Aluminum in large and small volume parenterals used in total parenteral nutrition. https://ecfr.io/cgi-bin/text-idx?SID=f2eed24e14658065465c1a54dd9eff04&mc=true&node=se21.4.201_1323&rgn=div8 Accessed 01 Jun 2020.
[123] AIT Institute. Aluminum Toxicity. https://www.aitinstitute.org/aluminum_toxicity.htm Accessed 01 Jun 2020.
[124] Ianelli V. Baby Birth Weight Statistics. VeryWell Family.Updated 29 Jun 2020. https://www.verywellfamily.com/baby-birth-weight-statistics-2633630#:~:text=The%20mean%20or%20average%20birth%20weight%20in%20the,grams%29%20is%20consider ed%20normal%20for%20a%20full-term%20newborn. Accessed 11 Sept 2020.
[125] Krewski, D., Yokel, R. A., Nieboer, E., Borchelt, D., Cohen, J., Harry, J., Kacew, S., Lindsay, J., Mahfouz, A. M., & Rondeau, V. (2007). Human health risk assessment for aluminium, aluminium oxide, and aluminium

clear toxins from their systems much more easily than children. A child's liver is not fully developed when he is born; rapid development continues to occur throughout the first year of life and toxin metabolism does not peak until the child is old enough to attend school.[126] In addition to the liver, the microbiome plays a major role in the elimination of toxic compounds from the body.[127] The composition of specific microbes in an individual's microbiome fluctuates a great deal in the first year of life, and it is likely that toxic assaults during this time may influence an individual throughout his lifetime.[128]

Additional studies have shown that the particular aluminum compounds used as adjuvants can persist in the body for *up to 11 years post-vaccination*,[129] which indicates that damage can continue to occur in children's bodies for at least a decade after receiving a vaccine. Due to this factor, the cumulative dosage of the adjuvant over an 11-year period should play an important role in determining whether the number of vaccines given on the CDC schedule is actually safe.

Unfortunately, bioaccumulation of aluminum is not the worst of the story when it comes to adjuvants. Studies done in mice show that these compounds are easily able to cross the blood-brain barrier, and accumulate in the brain, liver, spleen, and lymph nodes.[130] The ability to permeate into the central nervous system is especially troubling due to the neurotoxic effects of aluminum in the human body.[131] The risk of damage is much higher in infants and young children, who have a more permeable blood-brain barrier than older children and adults.[132]

In addition to the potential to cause severe neurological damage, aluminum adjuvants may also cause problems with the immune system. Because of the way that the adjuvant triggers the antibody response (bypassing the natural progression of immune activation in the body and shifting immunity away from a cellular response), it is possible that exposure to adjuvants can result in a long-term shift in how the body responds to pathogens.[133] This shift away from cell-mediated immunity can leave the body more susceptible to viral pathogens and to cancer. It has even been suggested that adjuvants play a role in mediating the development of allergic reactions, as the process of triggering allergic reactions is adjuvant-dependent.[134] This will be discussed in greater detail in a later section.

hydroxide. *Journal of toxicology and environmental health. Part B, Critical reviews*, *10 Suppl 1*(Suppl 1), 1–269. https://doi.org/10.1080/10937400701597766.

[126] Piñeiro-Carrero VM, Piñeiro EO. Liver. *Pediatrics* 2004 Apr, 113 (Supplement 3): 1097-1106.

[127] Murphy K, Travers P, Walport M. *Janeway's Immunobiology, 9th Ed.* New York and London: Garland Science, Taylor & Francis Group, 2017, p. 520.

[128] Gensollen T, Iyer SS, Kasper DL, Blumberg, RS. How colonization by microbiota in early life shapes the immune system. *Science.* 2016 April 29; 352(6285): 539–544. doi:10.1126/science.aad9378.

[129] Moskowitz, Richard MD. *Vaccines: A Reappraisal.* New York: Skyhorse Publishing, 2017, p, p. 79.

[130] Ibid, p. 164.

[131] Miller, Neil Z. *Miller's Review of Critical Vaccine Studies.* Santa Fe: New Atlantean Press, 2016, p. 44-61.

[132] Moskowitz, Richard MD. *Vaccines: A Reappraisal.* New York: Skyhorse Publishing, 2017, p.165.

[133] Tomljenovic L, Shaw C. Aluminum Vaccine Adjuvants: Are They Safe? *Cur Medicinal Chem* 2011, 18:2630.

[134] Obukhanych, T. *Vaccine Illusion.* Amazon Digital Services LLC, 2012.

# Vaccination and the Evolutionary Paradigm

*Again and again, faith in the truth of the evolutionary hypothesis has led scientists to see dysfunction or loss of function where there was functionality [...] This assumption of dysfunction in nature goes against the traditional presumption in favor of function that has characterized the pursuit of knowledge in medicine and natural science in the development of Western civilization.*
*--Hugh Owen[135]*

If the antibody model is defunct and the induction of immunity from vaccination is seriously limited, why is this medical intervention still perceived as a realistic option for managing the immune response?  One integral – and overlooked – reason is that vaccination is rooted in the modern evolutionary understanding of medicine.  This worldview ultimately reduces the body to a random amalgamation of factors that can effectively be tinkered with by man, who is considered more intelligent than his random maker, natural selection.  Before we discuss the specifics of vaccine safety and ethics, it is crucial to understand the foundations of evolutionary theory upon which the vaccine ideal rests.

## *The Creation-Providence Framework vs. the Evolutionary Paradigm*

From the beginning, the pioneers of vaccination focused on developing vaccines to combat or prevent specific diseases rather than striving to understand the human body's immune system or the ways that the body's natural defenses could be strengthened.  The preoccupation with specific diseases and with eliciting a specific response from the human body to those diseases reflects the Enlightenment philosophy of naturalism that came to dominate scientific and medical research during the late eighteenth and early nineteenth centuries.  Naturalism, which excludes any kind of supernatural cause and focuses on purely natural causes, logically leads to a reductionist interpretation of natural phenomena.  This, in turn, leads to practical consequences like the myopic focus on a single target molecule in the human body in order to treat disease symptoms, which is (quite unfortunately) the course of action pursued almost exclusively in modern drug development.[136]  We see this reductionism in its relation to vaccination most clearly evident in the idea that antibodies could be considered equivalent to immunity.

The philosophy of naturalism is incompatible with the faith of earlier natural scientists and doctors who believed in the special creation of man by an all-wise Creator.  Naturalism is based upon an evolutionary view of man (or at least of man's body, in the case of those who advocated a theistic version of evolution) as the product of undirected natural processes over long periods of time.  In light of this philosophy, man comes to be viewed as an "accident" – and despite his accidental nature, his attribute of intelligence becomes all-important in "fixing" whatever is wrong in the body and in the world.  The idea that man can substantially improve upon nature entered into its heyday with the eugenics movement that began in the late 1800s in England.  At that time, natural scientists worked to "improve" the genetics of crop plants, animals (especially dogs), and even

---

[135] Owen H. The negative impact of the evolutionary hypothesis on scientific research. 4 Feb 2010. https://kolbecenter.org/negative-impact-of-evolutionary-hypothesis-on-scientific-research/ Accessed 16 May 2020.
[136] Scapozza L. Drug Development. 2013. In: Global Health: An Interdisciplinary Overview. Coursera. https://www.coursera.org/learn/global-health-overview/lecture/6PxzP/drug-development-by-leonardo-scapozza Accessed 18 May 2020.

humans, using rigorous programs of selective breeding that pushed organisms to the limits of their genetic variability.* While the term eugenics has since acquired negative connotations and fallen out of favor, we can still see the arrogance of this mindset in examples such as research that is being done to genetically modify our food supply in order to make it sufficiently nutritious.[137,138] This is carried out despite the wealth of research that indicates that eating a variety of foods (as God created them) is more than adequate to meet human nutritional needs, and also in spite of concerns about the safety of genetically-modified food sources.[139] We also see this idea of man "making up for what is lacking" in creation when we consider that vaccines are designed to manipulate the body in an attempt to make the immune system more robust than it would be without them.

When evaluating the merits and demerits of vaccination, it is important to recognize that there are two different frameworks for doing scientific and medical research that have been used by notable researchers during the past few centuries. One framework is called the Creation-Providence Framework. This framework holds that Almighty God created the first human beings, Adam and Eve, instantly and without intermediate agents. They were perfect in body and mind, and free from any defect. The form of all living things is thus presumed to be stable in this framework, following the form created by God in the beginning, and all parts of God's creation are presumed to be functional, as all that God created is good. It was the Original Sin of Adam that brought death, deformity, and disease into the world, and these things were not an original part of creation; nor was death an integral part of the process by which living things were brought into being, as evolution theory supposes. Finally, sin damaged man *without destroying the essential goodness (and functionality) of the human body,* even as it is subject to death and decay.

This framework does not rest solely on a proper interpretation of Genesis, but also upon the work of one of the greatest of the Greek scientists and philosophers. In the Middle Ages, through the work of the Scholastic philosophers and theologians, the philosophy of Aristotle was thoroughly incorporated into the intellectual activity of the Church. According to Aristotle, everything in nature can be understood in terms of the four causes: material, efficient, formal, and final. These causes form an integral whole in explaining the purpose and nature of everything within living bodies.

The Creation-Providence framework heavily influenced such men as Francis Bacon and Sir William Harvey. Bacon is credited with developing the scientific method, which serves as the

---

* These programs of selective breeding that aimed to produce extremely "pure" bloodlines ultimately negatively impacted the health of the populations on which they were practiced. This was through the mechanism of reducing the overall variability of the gene pool, which rendered purebred organisms susceptible to various genetic defects that were accidentally bred into them alongside the more desirable characteristics. As we will see in many of the topics covered under vaccine safety (particularly with allergies, autoimmune reactions, and the shifting susceptibility of disease), there are also unintended side effects of the equally dangerous practice of trying to "engineer" the immune system.

[137] Haslam RP, Ruiz-Lopez N, Eastmond P, et al. The modification of plant oil composition via metabolic engineering—better nutrition by design. *Plant Biotechnology Journal,* 2013; 11, p. 157–168. doi: 10.1111/pbi.12012

[138] Le DT, Chu HD, Le NQ. Improving Nutritional Quality of Plant Proteins Through Genetic Engineering. *Curr Genomics.* 2016;17(3):220-229. doi:10.2174/1389202917666160202215934
These are only a few of the many examples that could be proffered.

[139] For more information on the tragedy of GMOs being introduced into the food supply, see: Owen H. *GMO Food: Boon or Bane?,* 2013. Published by author.

foundation for all empirical research in modern times. He definitively asserted the unity between truth in Scripture and truth in the observable world, thus maintaining the harmony between theology (the queen of the sciences) and natural science.[140] This framework also unquestionably drove Harvey in his quest to understand the circulation of the blood in the body.[141] He applied the principle that God works all things for a purpose, and that there was unity in the diversity of His designs. Harvey ultimately came to understand the circulation of the blood through analogy with other works of creation and their purpose.[142] These two men were not alone in their fruitful use of the Creation-Providence framework: this is the worldview that inspired many of the greatest minds in natural science, including Michael Faraday, James Joule, Blessed Nicholas Steno, Carolus Linneaus, George Washington Carver, and James Clerk Maxwell.

However, with the advent of Cartesian philosophy during the so-called Enlightenment, the subject of human origins was, without good reason, reassigned from the domain of theology to natural science and this soon required viewing mankind solely in terms of material and efficient causes—things that can be weighed, measured, and quantified. This was truly tragic, for modern biologists recognize that function follows form, and they recognize the importance of understanding the structure to understand the function of living things and their organs and organ systems. This recognition implies that *specific forms are required for specific purposes*; however, modern biologists must presume that all these functional forms *do not serve a purpose* (i.e. do not have a final cause) if they follow their philosophy whole-heartedly. And it cannot truly be followed whole-heartedly, for even the most committed materialists among them fail to completely eradicate the idea of purposiveness from their language.

By embracing naturalistic uniformitarianism, adherents to what we might call the evolutionary framework no longer presume stable form and function throughout the biosphere, but instead presume flux and dysfunction. Natural scientists imbued with materialism no longer look at plants or animals as integrated, created wholes but as collections of parts, like machines, that could be cobbled together bit by bit over long ages of time. Moreover, the assembly of these living machines is held to be random and the result of genetic errors (mutations).

This framework, which preceded Darwin and flowed from the Cartesian philosophy of rationalism, appears to have been shared by Edward Jenner and the other pioneers of vaccination. The presumption that without vaccination the body will be unable to face the regular onslaught of pathogens in its environment (the body is randomly assembled, and so human reason must be able to "improve" upon its design and thus its function) and the idea that we could manipulate only a part of the immune system without producing possible unintended effects in the body as a whole (since the body is an arbitrary assemblage of parts that may be adjusted individually and unsystematically) are both of a piece with this evolutionary framework.

Vaccination is not the first time that naturalism has imposed itself on medicine through the impoverished evolutionary paradigm. The reductionist view of plants and animals also led to the perverse conviction that organs or features of plants, animals, or humans that had no apparent

---

[140] Morris HM. Sir Francis Bacon. 16 Feb 1998. https://answersingenesis.org/creation-scientists/profiles/sir-francis-bacon/ Accessed 18 May 2020.
[141] Bergman J. The ends justify the means – The secret of science's success. *J Creation*, 2013; 27(1): 19-22.
[142] Ibid.

function were "useless" vestigial leftovers from an earlier stage of a long natural evolutionary process. This fit neatly within the framework of evolutionary organs, and the reductionist idea that bodies were assemblages of disconnected parts. It would prove to have several disastrous consequences.

It was originally claimed by evolutionary scientists that up to 180 organs in the human body were vestigial.[143] As this belief in vestigial organs entered the mainstream of scientific and medical training, medical researchers grew even more likely to presume flux and dysfunction in the plants, animals, and humans they studied. Worse still, in opposition to Harvey, researchers began to assume that what they did not understand was a result of random chance. Lacking a framework with final causes, they did not search for a purpose or use for that which they did not understand. As a result, medical and scientific investigation departed from the full truth about mankind and dangerous and unnecessary practices were perpetuated. It is important to give a brief history of this idea of "vestigiality," with specific examples of its impact on medical progress, to illustrate the depth and consequences of embracing the evolutionary framework as the basis for medical interventions.

### Tonsils: Vestigial Organs or Vanguards of the Mucosal Immune System?

For many decades, the tonsils were classified as vestigial organs and routinely removed unnecessarily from millions of patients. Only in the recent past were doctors and medical researchers forced to recognize that tonsils are an integral part of the human immune system[144] and that tonsil removal actually amounted to stripping patients of part of their God-given first line of immune defense. Reports from doctors during the polio epidemics of the mid-twentieth century confirmed that patients who had had their tonsils removed were far more likely than those who kept their tonsils to suffer the worst effects of the disease.[145] Long-term studies have further demonstrated that individuals who did not have their tonsils removed were comparably healthier after thirty years than those who did.[146]

It is reasonable to conclude that a large percentage (and probably the vast majority) of the tens of thousands of patients who died as a result of a tonsillectomy, as well as the hundreds of thousands who suffered complications requiring hospitalization,[147] should never have had the operation at all. But the evolutionary presumption that the tonsils were vestigial – that they developed through random natural processes and served no purpose in the human body – was also dangerous for another reason. It shifted attention away from the physiological and environmental factors responsible for the swelling of the tonsils (which in turn led to chronic infection or blocked airways) and pinned the blame for these conditions on an assumed defect in the "vestigial" tonsils themselves.

---

[143] *The World's Most Famous Court Trial*, second reprint edition, Bryan College, Dayton, Tennessee, 1990, p. 228.
[144] Seladi-Schulman J. Tonsils and Adenoids Overview. https://www.healthline.com/health/tonsils-and-adenoids#function (accessed 4-22-20)
[145] *Time* magazine, "Tonsils & Bulbar Polio," Monday, Apr. 12, 1954.
[146] Van Staaji B, van den Akker FH, Rovers MM, Hordijk GJ, Hoes AW, Schilder AGM. Effectiveness of adenotonsillectomy in children with mild symptoms of throat infections or adenotonsillar hypertrophy: open, randomised controlled trial. *British Medical Journal*, 2004 Sept 18: 329-651. doi:10.1136/bmj.38210.827917.7C
[147] A study of complications from tonsillectomy in England and Scotland discovered a rate of 2-5% in 2000-2001 http://www.entuk.org/audits/reporttonsillectomysurvey_pdf

Adherence to the evolutionary hypothesis has made it more difficult for medical researchers to explore the possibility that the swelling of the tonsils in relation to the air passage might be related to problems with diet, environment, and lifestyle. These factors can result in the under-development of the bony structures that house the tonsils, and so the blocked airways may not be indicative of any kind of dysfunction in the tonsils themselves. Orthodontist Dr. Raymond Silkman notes that:

> "[…] the soft tissues of the body grow to their genetic size, even when the bony structures do not. The skin, the tongue, the tonsils and the nasal tissues grow to their genetic size but when the nutrition is missing, the bony structures are compromised. So the face will have an excess of skin and musculature, the tongue and tonsils will be too large for the mouth […]."[148]

In modern times, the primary reason for the hundreds of thousands of tonsillectomies performed each year is blockage of the airway.[149] If Dr. Silkman is correct, these tonsillectomies will continue to treat the symptom (the enlarged tonsils) instead of the cause (environmental pollution, lack of exercise and malnutrition) by removing a part of the patients' already compromised immune system. This not only exposes the patient to unnecessary risk, but will likely negatively impact the body's ability to deal with the factors that caused the problem in the first place.

Since this paper focuses on the scientific merits and demerits of vaccination, one additional example is sufficient to illustrate the harmful role that the all-but-universal acceptance of the evolutionary hypothesis has had in preventing an objective evaluation of the scientific basis for vaccination. Our second example involves the human appendix.

### *The Vermiform Appendix: Useless Appendage or Vital Organ of the Immune System?*

Darwin held that the appendix was vestigial because it was small in comparison with the caecum* of monkeys. This smallness was represented as evidence that in the course of man's evolution the need for the caecum had diminished as his diet had changed; the result was that the caecum and the appendix (or caecal appendage) had grown smaller in man through "disuse."[150] Acceptance of the evolutionary hypothesis by most biologists and medical researchers ensured that the actual function of the appendix in humans remained obscure for over a century after *Origin of Species*.[151]

---

[148] Silkman R. Is it Mental or is it Dental? Cranial & Dental Impacts on Total Health. http://www.westonaprice.org/healthissues/facial-development.html Accessed 08 March 2009.

[149] Mayo Clinic. Tonsillectomy. 2010 Nov 10. www.mayoclinic.org/tests-procedures/tonsillectomy/about/pac-20395141. Accessed 2020 Nov 14.

* The caecum is a small pouch connected to the junction of the small and large intestines.

[150] Darwin C. *The Descent of Man*. 2nd ed. 1874, chap. 1, http://bibliotecadigital.puc-campinas.edu.br/services/e-books/Charles%20Darwin-1.pdf (accessed 4-22-20).

[151] Perkel A, Needleman MH: *Biology for All*. New York: Barnes and Noble, 1950, p. 129.

However, in the 1960's, experimental evidence demonstrated that the appendix actually serves as a center for antibody-producing cells.[152] By 1976, experimental knowledge of the appendix "evolved" to the point that a medical textbook on gastroenterology noted the following:

> The appendix is not generally credited with significant function; however, current evidence tends to involve it in the immunologic mechanism.[153]

Further research demonstrated that the appendix is part of the Gut Associated Lymphoid Tissue system (or G.A.L.T.) which produces several kinds of antibodies: IgA immunoglobulins, which help to protect the bloodstream from infection from the contents of the bowel, and IgM and IgG immunoglobulins, which combat infections in the bloodstream.[154] In 1995, a textbook on anatomy and physiology stated categorically that:

> The mucosa and submucosa of the appendix are dominated by lymphoid nodules, and its primary function is as an organ of the lymphatic system.[155]

It is now recognized that the lymphoid nodules appear in the appendix roughly two weeks after birth, which coincides with the colonization of the bowel with bacteria.[156] We also now know that there is an important interplay between the appendix and the microbiome, and that its impact on health is much more complex than was first realized.[157]

In spite of the overwhelming evidence for the functionality of the appendix, 150 years after *Origin of Species*, Darwin's dim view of the organ continues to be upheld by respected information sources. For example, as late as 2009, a visitor to the British Broadcasting Corporation's "Science and Nature Home Page" could still read the following description of the appendix:

> The appendix has no known function in humans. Evidence suggests that our evolutionary ancestors used their appendixes to digest tough food like tree bark, but we don't use ours in digestion now. Some scientists believe that the appendix will disappear from the human body.[158]

The extraordinary ignorance of this statement shows how much faith in the evolutionary hypothesis continues to influence leaders in the field of public information, even when the facts contradict their presuppositions. On another note, the statement also reflects the degree to which the conventional wisdom pins the blame for diseases of the appendix squarely on the "vestigial"

---

[152] https://creation.com/the-human-vermiform-appendix (accessed 4-22-20)

[153] McHardy G: chap. "The Appendix". In: Bockus HL. (ed.): *Gastroenterology* 1976; 2: 1134-1148.

[154] Glover JW. The human vermiform appendix. *Journal of Creation* (formerly TJ) 1998 April; 3(1):31–38 https://creation.com/the-human-vermiform-appendix Accessed 22 April 2020.

[155] Martini FH.: *Fundamentals of Anatomy and Physiology*. Englewood Cliffs, NJ: Prentice Hall, 1995, p. 916.

[156] Glover JW. The human vermiform appendix. *Journal of Creation* (formerly TJ) 1998 April; 3(1):31–38 https://creation.com/the-human-vermiform-appendix Accessed 22 April 2020.

[157] Guinane CM, Tadrous A, Fouhy F, et al. Microbial composition of human appendices from patients following appendectomy. *mBio*. 2013;4(1):e00366-12. Published 2013 Jan 15. doi:10.1128/mBio.00366-12

[158] British Broadcasting Corporation. Science and Nature Home Page, "Science: Human Body and Mind" http://www.bbc.co.uk/science/humanbody/body/factfiles/appendix/appendix.shtml Accessed 11 December 2020.

and defective nature of the organ itself, without even considering the possibility that these diseases could be symptomatic of deeper disorders.

By conducting an extensive study of non-modernized societies all over the world, Dr. Weston Price found that appendicitis was virtually non-existent in those who retained their traditional diet and way of life. Typical was the testimony of Dr. Romig who lived among the non-modernized Eskimos of Alaska and who stated that:

> in his thirty-six years of contact with these people he had never seen a case of malignant disease among the truly primitive Eskimos and Indians, although it frequently occurs when they become modernized. He found, similarly, that the acute surgical problems requiring operation on internal organs, such as the gall bladder, kidney, stomach and appendix, do not tend to occur among the primitives but are very common problems among the modernized Eskimos and Indians.[159]

By blaming diseases of the appendix on the "defective condition" of a "vestigial organ," the evolutionary framework has helped to discourage researchers from following the traditional approach of Western natural science and medical research. This approach looked for the causes of human disease in the defective diet, habits, or environment of their patients rather than in some intrinsic defect of the body or of its component parts. By blaming diseases of a vestigial appendix on evolutionary factors, generations of scientists have lost their incentive to ask why these diseases did not exist among non-industrialized societies and to seek to prevent them through constructive changes in diet and life-style rather than by treating the symptoms of the disease through surgical removal. This idea of alternative ways of dealing with disease symptoms will be addressed again at the close of this work, as it plays an important role in decision-making regarding vaccination.

## The Brilliant Blindness of Evolution-Based Medicine

Mainstream medicine's approach to the tonsils and the vermiform appendix suffice to demonstrate that brilliant scientists and medical researchers go astray when they embrace the naturalistic evolutionary framework. The framework was the primary reason that generations of brilliant researchers failed to investigate the vital role of the tonsils and the appendix in the immune system. The current global trend to seek a vaccine for every contagious disease—while weakening the overall strength and integrity of the body's immune system through the introduction of disease agents and toxins directly into the bloodstream—represents an intensification of the application of the errors of this framework to the treatment of disease. The falsification of the myth of vestigial organs and their role in disease pathology ought to serve as a warning that the global promotion of vaccination as a key to eradicating disease needs to be reevaluated. It also ought to inspire a return to the Creation-Providence framework of St. Albert the Great, Sir William Harvey, and the great scientific and medical researchers of the pre-Enlightenment period.

---

[159] Price WA. *Nutrition and Physical Degeneration*, La Mesa, 2000, p. 91.
For more information on this hypothesis, see: Burkitt DP. The Aetiology of Appendicitis. *British Journal of Surgery*, 1971; 58(9) 695-699.

With this framework in mind, we will return to our examination of vaccines, and to a thorough assessment of their safety and the moral and ethical issues that accompany current vaccination policy.

# The Safety of Vaccination

*Despite the huge amount of money invested in studying vaccines,*
*there are few observational studies and virtually no randomized clinical trials documenting*
*the effect on mortality of any of the existing vaccines.*
*-- ASIA study authors*[160]

Even if vaccines are not natural, wholly effective, or based in sound principles of basic science, most vaccines are accompanied by a moderate, short-term reduction in the disease they are designed to prevent. Therefore, a reasonable argument could be made for continuing some sort of mass vaccination policy if vaccines were at least demonstrably safe. However, there is evidence that individual vaccines (particularly DTaP, HPV, and the influenza vaccine) result in unacceptable rates of adverse reactions, some of which are severe or even life-threatening. A host of questions have also been raised about individual ingredients in the vaccines – ranging from heavy metals to detergents to aborted fetal tissue contaminants – that cast additional doubt on the safety of particular vaccines. Even the process of vaccination itself has been implicated as possibly (or even probably) harmful, as it is able to induce aberrations of the immune system like autoimmune disease and allergies. Each of these concerns is sufficient to raise alarm on its own, but when combined, the case can readily be made that the risk of injury from vaccination is unacceptably high. This chapter will address all of these specific cases against vaccine safety, and will also cover problems that result at a population level from mandatory mass vaccination. These problems include the rise of new strains of pathogens as well as the substitution of chronic disease for infectious disease.

## *Contraindications for Vaccines*

While often cited as providing ample assurance that vaccines are both safe and effective, the Centers for Disease Control and Prevention (CDC)* gives a long list of conditions that make it unadvisable for individuals to receive each of the licensed vaccines. The table below lists these conditions, known as contraindications, for all the vaccines currently recommended on the CDC schedule from birth to 18 years. Definite contraindications are conditions that should certainly prevent an individual from being vaccinated, because he could potentially risk his life if these conditions are present; possible contraindications are conditions that warrant additional caution but may not be as serious as definite contraindications (though they may still be linked to adverse

---

[160] Perricone C, Colafrancesco S, et al. Autoimmune/inflammatory syndrome induced by adjuvants (ASIA) 2013: Unveiling the pathogenic, clinical and diagnostic aspects. *Journal of Autoimmunity*, 2013; 47: 1-16. http://dx.doi.org/10.1016/j.jaut.2013.10.004

* According to MedicineNet (https://www.medicinenet.com/script/main/art.asp?articlekey=2655), the CDC is "the US agency charged with tracking and investigating public health trends. A part of the US Public Health Services (PHS) under the Department of Health and Human Services (HHS), the CDC is based in Atlanta, Georgia. It publishes key health information, including weekly data on all deaths and diseases reported in the US and travelers' health advisories. The CDC also fields special rapid-response teams to halt epidemic diseases." The CDC's own mission statement says that the CDC "works 24/7 to protect America from health, safety and security threats, both foreign and in the U.S. Whether diseases start at home or abroad, are chronic or acute, curable or preventable, human error or deliberate attack, CDC fights disease and supports communities and citizens to do the same." Because of the nature and status of this organization, many people place a great deal of trust in the agency's pronouncements on medical matters.

effects). A life–threatening allergy to any component of the vaccine is a definite contraindication of all vaccines; vaccines should never be given to individuals who have such allergies.

| Vaccine | Definite Contraindications | Possible Contraindications |
|---|---|---|
| Hepatitis B (Birth[161]) | – a life-threatening reaction to the Hepatitis A vaccine | – any illness |
| Rotavirus (2 months) | – a life-threatening allergic reaction to a prior dose of vaccine <br> – severe combined immuno-deficiency disorder (SCID) <br> – an intussecption (a kind of obstruction of the bowel) | – HIV/AIDS <br> – cancer <br> – taking medication that affects the immune system |
| Diphtheria (2 months) | – a serious reaction to any diphtheria, pertussis, or tetanus vaccine | – seizures <br> – any other neurological illness <br> – serious pain or swelling after any diphtheria, pertussis, or tetanus vaccine <br> – Guillain-Barré Syndrome |
| Tetanus (2 months) | – a serious reaction to any diphtheria, pertussis, or tetanus vaccine | – seizures <br> – any other neurological illness <br> – serious pain or swelling after any diphtheria, pertussis, or tetanus vaccine <br> – Guillain-Barré Syndrome |
| Pertussis (whooping cough) (2 months) | – a serious reaction to any diphtheria, pertussis, or tetanus vaccine | – seizures <br> – any other neurological illness <br> – serious pain or swelling after any diphtheria, pertussis, or tetanus vaccine <br> – Guillain-Barré Syndrome |
| Hib (2 months) | – a life-threatening allergic reaction to a prior dose of vaccine <br> – a serious allergy to any component of the vaccine <br> – children younger than 6 weeks | |
| Pneumococcal (2 months) | – a life-threatening allergic reaction to a prior dose of vaccine | – serious allergies of any kind <br> – pregnancy |
| Polio (2 months) | – a life-threatening allergic reaction to a prior dose of vaccine | – any serious allergies <br> – any illness |
| Influenza (IM) (6 months) | – an allergy to gelatin or neomycin <br> – age younger than 6 months | – Guillain-Barré Syndrome <br> – any illness |
| MMR (measles, mumps, and rubella) (12 months) | – a life-threatening allergic reaction to a prior dose of vaccine <br> – pregnancy | – HIV/AIDS <br> – cancer <br> – low platelet count <br> – taking medication that affects the immune system <br> – receiving another vaccine within 30 days <br> – recent blood transfusion |

---

[161] All ages in the table are taken from The Centers for Disease Control, *Table 1. Recommended Child and Adolescent Immunization Schedule for ages 18 years or younger*, United States, 2019. https://www.cdc.gov/vaccines/schedules/hcp/imz/child-adolescent.html Accessed 11 Sept 2019.

| Vaccine | Definite Contraindications | Possible Contraindications |
|---|---|---|
| Varicella (Chickenpox) (12 months) | – an allergy to gelatin or neomycin<br>– a blood transfusion within the past 11 months<br>– a current illness more serious than a cold | – any immune system disorder<br>– taking medication that affects the immune system<br>– receiving treatment for cancer |
| Hepatitis A (12 months) | – a life-threatening allergy to any component of the vaccine | – any illness |
| HPV (9-12 years) | – a life-threatening allergic reaction to a prior dose of vaccine | – pregnancy<br>– any serious allergies, including to yeast |
| Meningococcal (11-12 years) | – a life-threatening allergic reaction to a prior dose of vaccine | – serious allergies of any kind<br>– pregnancy<br>– breastfeeding |

**Table 2: Contraindication of Vaccines**[162]

As can be seen from this list, even the CDC acknowledges many documented instances where vaccines are unsafe. Yet individuals are generally not screened for these conditions prior to vaccination, and some states have even recently passed laws that make obtaining medical exemptions to vaccination difficult even for those who truly need them.[163] It is noteworthy that the US Department of Health and Human Services recommends against receiving a vaccine in any case where the individual has a serious allergic reaction to either the active or inactive ingredients of the vaccine, or to any vaccine for a similar pathogen; *yet the CDC recommends that all children receive the majority of these vaccines before it would be possible to determine whether they had any allergies at all.* This policy leads to a situation in which it is impossible to know whether most individuals display contraindications for vaccination until it is too late and they have experienced an adverse reaction to one or more vaccine components.

It is also important to note that many vaccines have "any illness" listed as a contraindication. In situations where policies have made vaccines unavoidable, as with military personnel or hospital employees, it is important to know that even slight illnesses, such as head colds, should be an occasion to reschedule a vaccination appointment.

### *Trading One Disease for Another: Adverse Vaccine Reactions*

In 2011, a US Supreme Court Ruling (Bruesewitz v. Wyeth) determined that vaccines qualify as products that are "unavoidably unsafe."[164] This is defined as any products which "in the present state of human knowledge, are quite incapable of being made safe for their intended and ordinary use."[165] Thus, *vaccine manufacturers are exempt from liability* in the event that a disability or death results from the use of their product. While the phrase "unavoidably unsafe" is a legal designation rather than a scientific one, the list of possible adverse side effects from vaccines is long, and does include seriously debilitating and life-threatening events.

---

[162] All information taken from individual vaccine pages at Vaccine.Gov (U.S. Department of Health & Human Services): https://www.vaccines.gov/diseases Accessed 11 Sept 2019.

[163] CalMatters. "Five things to know now about California's new vaccine law." 15 Sept 2019. https://calmatters.org/health/2019/09/california-new-law-vaccination-medical-exemption/ Accessed 28 Oct 2019.

[164] Supreme Court of the United States. Russell Bruesewitz, et al. v. Wyeth LLC, Wyeth, Inc, Wyeth Laboratories, et al. 22 Feb 2011. https://www.law.cornell.edu/supct/html/09-152.ZD.html Accessed 18 May 2020.

[165] Ibid.

Unfortunately, many of these reactions and side effects are dismissed out of hand as being unrelated to the vaccine.* Parents report that when they mention the possibility of a connection between a vaccine and the onset of new and serious changes in their child, they are often immediately told that there is no connection, sometimes almost before they can get the question out of their mouths.• However, as parents are generally the best judge of changes in normal behavior for their children, and likely to be very sensitive as to the nature and timing of these changes, it seems absurd to dismiss out-of-hand their judgment that their child was progressing normally until just after a recent vaccination.

A national reporting system for vaccine reactions exists, but it suffers from some significant limitations. The Vaccine Adverse Events Reporting System, or VAERS, website states that it allows physicians, parents, or the patients themselves to report any "clinically important adverse events" that follow a vaccination.[166] Since the data is self-reported, it is estimated that only 1-10% of adverse reactions to vaccines are actually submitted to VAERS.[167] This fact alone would make it difficult to use VAERS data to determine anything significant about the safety of vaccinations, but it is further complicated by the fact that many of the conditions that could potentially be caused by vaccines (such as autism, autoimmune disorders, allergies, ADHD, and other chronic conditions) may not have an immediate temporal link to the time of the vaccination, and so it is more unlikely that they will be reported to the system. Many also point out that since VAERS does not make a determination regarding whether the adverse event was or was not causally connected with the vaccine, there is little utility in using such statistics; some even go so far as to suggest that non-causal reports balance out the non-reported events in such a way that the incidence of serious side effects (such as disability or death) is as low as one might gather from the VAERS raw data.[168] However, there are also vaccine proponents who point to VAERS as an important tool for post-licensing safety data, even going so far as to say that it is "essential to determine whether the safety profiles established in prelicensing studies are reflected during use in the general population, and to detect previously unrecognized or rare adverse events."[169]

Dr. Robert Sears cites a 1991-2001 study by the CDC on VAERS data that reports an incidence of severe adverse reactions (which the CDC describes as "a prolonged hospital stay, a severe life-threatening illness, a permanent disability, or death") as around 1 serious adverse event per 100,000 doses of vaccine. However, this data is now nearly 20 years old, and in the decade after the data was published the vaccine schedule doubled and the VAERS reports increased by slightly

---

* Only 0.4% of the serious adverse reactions reported by patients during clinical testing of the vaccine Gardasil® were accepted as being related to the vaccine. 99.6% of the reactions were dismissed and so did not affect the conclusion of the study. This is only one example among many of how vaccine proponents ignore substantial evidence of vaccine harm. (Moskowitz, 2017, p 32)

• Readers are encouraged to view the documentaries *The Greater Good*, *Vaxxed*, and *Vaxxed II* for many examples of this phenomenon. *Vaxxed* also has a YouTube channel where many more parents have been interviewed and shared their stories.

[166] VAERS. "Frequently Asked Questions." https://vaers.hhs.gov/faq.html Accessed 28 Oct 2019.

[167] Vernon LF. How Silencing of Dissent in Science Impacts Woman. The Gardasil® Story. *Advances in Sexual Medicine*, 2017; 7: 179-204. *See also:* references 92-94 from the same paper.

[168] Sears RW. *The Vaccine Book*. New York: Little, Brown and Company, 2011, p. 191-193.

[169] Roush SW, Murphy TV, et al. Historical Comparisons of Morbidity and Mortality for Vaccine-Preventable Diseases in the United States. *JAMA*, 2007 Nov 14; 298(18): 2155-2163.

more than two-fold.[170] Also, this statistic does not give an accurate picture of the overall risk per person, since each person receives significantly more than one dose of vaccine in his lifetime.* Dr. Sears breaks this risk down in a number of ways, but his assessment of infant risk is particularly interesting. Taking as a rough estimate that about half of vaccine doses are given to infants under the age of two, he also estimates that about half of the adverse reactions occur in this population. Then using the average number of infants born per year in the United States, he estimates a risk of adverse reactions to vaccination as 1 in 5,300 infants.[171] If this is adjusted to reflect the estimated rate of reporting of actual adverse reactions to the VAERS system, the incidence is probably closer to between 1 in 530 to 1 in 53 infants who experience a severe adverse reaction to a vaccination. If these numbers are even approximately accurate, this would suggest that the risks of vaccinating an infant far outweigh any possible benefits.

While Dr. Sears' estimates are very rough, and do not account for adverse reactions that are reported to VAERS which may not be caused by vaccines (which would lower the incidence of adverse events), they also do not account for the possible connection just mentioned between vaccines and long-term, slow-onset disorders like autoimmunity and allergies (which would likely significantly compound the problem). These two cases of vaccine-linked illnesses deserve a more in-depth examination, which will be undertaken in the next two sections.

## Trading One Disease for Another: Autoimmunity

As previously explained, the key function of the immune system is to distinguish that which is "self" from that which is "non-self" and to eliminate the latter from the body. The collection of cells and organs that works together to accomplish this is precisely and efficiently destructive. When the body's immune system is primed against a component of the body itself, it leads to the development of autoimmune disease. When the body's immune system is primed against a harmless environmental agent, it leads to the development of allergy. Both processes can result from vaccination – because vaccination is, by its very nature, the artificial activation of an intense immune response and it has been documented that this response is cross-reactive.[172] This cross-reactivity means that the body may be sensitized to multiple "antigens" from a single vaccine, and this may include parts of the body's own tissue, harmless additions to the vaccine like egg protein, or even foods that were recently consumed.

There is an extremely strong case that vaccines can trigger autoimmune diseases in susceptible individuals.[173] This is thought to be mediated particularly through exposure to the aluminum adjuvants that are present in subunit vaccines (as well as some inactivated vaccines), leading researchers to describe some autoimmune conditions as "autoimmune/inflammatory syndrome

[170] Sears RW. *The Vaccine Book.* New York: Little, Brown and Company, 2011, p. 191-193.
* The CDC schedule lists 33 recommended doses of vaccines for children up to 18 years of age (not counting the annual influenza vaccine), but as many of these are multivalent that number is somewhat misleading. If you include each of the separate vaccine components as its own dose, the number is closer to 49, plus an additional 17 doses of an annual influenza vaccine, for a total of at least 66 doses of vaccines.
[171] Ibid, p. 192.
[172] Benn CS, Netea MG, Selin LK, Peter A. A small jab – a big effect: nonspecific immunomodulation by vaccines. *Trends in Immunology*, 2013 May 14. http://dx.doi.org/10.1016/j.it.2013.04.004
[173] Miller NZ. *Miller's Review of Critical Vaccine Studies.* Santa Fe: New Atlantean Press, 2016. References 35-36, 39-46, 54-61, 154-159, 163, 175, 201, 205-211, 244-274.

induced by adjuvants" (ASIA).[174] The body has a natural "screening" process for immune cells in order to eliminate self-reactive cells, and this process eliminates nearly all of the cells that would attack the body itself.[175] However, the introduction of an adjuvant, along with the active component of the vaccine, creates abnormal immunological conditions by selectively activating and highly overstimulating some components of the immune system, and this may cause some self-reactive cells to slip through the cracks of the screening process.

This is not a hypothetical scenario. Animal studies have shown that the heightened immune activation that is produced by a vaccine adjuvant does cause some self-reactive immune cells to be activated. [176] The activation itself is temporary, common, and often quickly corrected by the immune system. However, since self-antigens are not cleared from the body the way that normal antigens are, if a self-reactive cell is allowed to replicate, the activation quickly turns into chronic disease. ** Chronic inflammation in affected tissues creates a positive feedback loop that heightens the pathology of the disorder by releasing more self-antigens as tissue continues to be damaged and also by recruiting more innate immune cells to the site of the inflammation.[177] It is particularly important to note that the vast majority, if not all, of autoimmune conditions are mediated by antibodies – which are precisely the same immune effectors that vaccination seeks to induce to an excessive extent. Indeed, self-reactive antibodies have been the litmus test for diagnosing autoimmune disorders from the time they began to be diagnosed.[178]

These disorders develop over extended periods of time, and the chronology of their development can be hard to characterize. We still know relatively little about just why prolonged reactions occur in certain individuals, rather than the short-term activation that is quickly cleared from the body, though there may be some genetic component involved. It can be very difficult to establish rigorous scientific causality regarding chronic autoimmune disease, and vaccine manufacturers and many researchers are generally reluctant to admit that there is a connection between vaccines and autoimmunity. This reluctance is despite the fact that a primary underlying mechanism of auto-reactivity has been causally associated with vaccines and nearly all types of vaccine have been associated with autoimmune onset in well-established case studies.[179]

---

[174] Shoenfeld Y, Agmon-Levin N. 'ASIA' – Autoimmune/inflammatory syndrome induced by adjuvants. *Journal of Autoimmunity,* 2011 Feb; 36(1): 4-8.

[175] Murphy K, Travers P, and Walport M. *Janeway's Immunobiology.* New York and London: Garland Science, Taylor & Francis Group, 2008, p. 258.

[176] Shoenfeld Y, Agmon-Levin N. 'ASIA' – Autoimmune/inflammatory syndrome induced by adjuvants. *Journal of Autoimmunity,* 2011 Feb; 36(1): 4-8.

** For readers who are interested in a more detailed explanation of the possible mechanism of the onset of post-vaccination autoimmune disorders than can be provided here, please see: Perricone C, Colafrancesco S, et al. Autoimmune/inflammatory syndrome induced by adjuvants (ASIA) 2013: Unveiling the pathogenic, clinical and diagnostic aspects. *Journal of Autoimmunity*, 47 (2013) 1-16. http://dx.doi.org/10.1016/j.jaut.2013.10.004

[177] Murphy K, Travers P, and Walport M. *Janeway's Immunobiology, 9th Ed.* New York and London: Garland Science, Taylor & Francis Group, 2017, p. 657-659.

[178] Johns Hopkins University. Definition of Autoimmunity & Autoimmune Disease. https://pathology.jhu.edu/autoimmune/definitions/ Accessed 18 May 2020.

[179] Perricone C, Colafrancesco S, et al. Autoimmune/inflammatory syndrome induced by adjuvants (ASIA) 2013: Unveiling the pathogenic, clinical and diagnostic aspects. *Journal of Autoimmunity*, 47 (2013) 1-16. http://dx.doi.org/10.1016/j.jaut.2013.10.004

Allergies are characterized by inappropriate activation of the immune system in the presence of a harmless antigen.[180] With the exception of contact dermatitis (the characteristic allergic rash that develops after exposure to a trigger like poison ivy), the majority of allergic reactions are mediated by antibodies. Once an individual has been "sensitized" to a very low dose of a particular antigen (dust, pollen, peanuts, or any one of many common allergens), his body reacts by producing large amounts of antibodies whenever there is a secondary exposure to the allergen, as well as recruiting other immune cells (mast cells and basophils) that launch the full blown immunological response that is characterized as an allergic reaction. [181]

Aluminum adjuvants are again the primary candidate for a biological mechanism to explain how vaccine exposure could induce allergies. The nature of the adjuvant is to heighten an immune response to a weak antigen, so it is not unreasonable to propose that if the vaccinated individual is exposed to some harmless antigen at a time when the adjuvant is circulating readily in his system, the presence of the adjuvant would help induce a response to the potential allergen as well as to the vaccine components.

Not only is the mechanism plausible, but a number of studies have reported statistically significant results in the association of vaccines with the development of allergic diseases, including the following:

   – MMR and DPT vaccines are associated with the development of asthma and eczema.[182]
   – Pertussis vaccines are associated with asthma, hay fever and food allergies.[183]
   – Of a sample of 1,265 children in New Zealand who received the DPT and polio vaccines, 30% underwent consultations for allergic illness.[184]
   – Delaying vaccination for pertussis reduces the risk of developing asthma.[185]
   – Delaying vaccination for pertussis, measles-mumps-rubella, or tuberculosis reduces the risk of developing hay fever.[186]

While correlation does not necessarily imply causation, these associations should give pause to those who assert that there is no connection between vaccines and allergies. In addition, the fact that anaphylaxis (the most severe, life-threatening allergic reaction) is a reportable adverse event

---

[180] Murphy K, Travers P, and Walport M. *Janeway's Immunobiology, 9th Ed.* New York and London: Garland Science, Taylor & Francis Group, 2017, p. 32-33.
[181] Ibid, p. 555-556.
[182] McKeever TM, Lewis SA, et al. Vaccination and allergic disease: a birth cohort study. *Am J Public Health* 2004 Jun; 94(6): 985-89.
[183] Bernsen RM, Nagelkerke NJ, et al. Reported pertussis infection and risk of atopy in 8- to 12-year-old vaccinated and non-vaccinated children. *Pediatr Allergy Immunol* 2008 Feb; 19(1): 46-52.
[184] Kemp T, Pearce N, et al. Is infant immunization a risk factor for childhood asthma or allergy? *Epidemiology* 1997 Nov; 8(6) 678-680.
[185] McDonald KL, Hu1 SI, et al. Delay in diphtheria, pertussis, tetanus vaccination is associated with a reduced risk of childhood asthma. *J Allergy Clin Immunol* 2008 Mar; 121(3): 626-31.
[186] Brmner SA, Carey IM, et al. Timing of routine immunization and subsequent hay fever risk. *Arch Dis Child* 2005; 90: 567-573.

that is recognized by VAERS* provides more evidence that vaccines are biologically plausible culprits in the induction of allergic reactions.[187]

## *Vaccines and Autism: Link or No Link?*

No paper on vaccination can remain silent regarding the alleged connection between vaccines and autism. Dr. Andrew Wakefield is generally credited as having first made this assertion in 1998, after examining eight children who developed gastrointestinal issues and developmental delays consistent with autism.[188] These symptoms were temporally related to the patients' receipt of a measles-mumps-rubella vaccine (MMR), and while Dr. Wakefield quickly became a center of controversy, the strongest statement he made in the paper was incredibly mild. He suggested only that the possibility of a link between the MMR vaccine and autism ought to be investigated:

> We did not prove an association between measles, mumps, and rubella vaccine and the syndrome described [autism]. Virological studies are underway that may help to resolve this issue. [189]

> If there is a causal link between measles, mumps, and rubella vaccine and this syndrome, a rising incidence might be anticipated after the introduction of this vaccine in the UK in 1988. Published evidence is inadequate to show whether there is a change in incidence or a link with measles, mumps, and rubella vaccine.[190]

In later testimony given before a congressional committee, he made no more controversial suggestion than that the measles, mumps, and rubella components of the vaccine be administered separately.[191] Despite the reasonableness of his statements, he quickly became the subject of investigations and personal attacks. The journal retracted his 1998 paper in 2004, and his medical license was revoked in 2010.[192] While a number of claims were made regarding the validity of his data, the only reason that the *Lancet* gave for the paper's retraction was an undisclosed conflict of interest with an entity called Legal Aid (from which Dr. Wakefield had received compensation for his work with the original eight children in the study).[193] To this date, no one has actually

---

* As a possible outcome of tetanus, pertussis, MMR, polio, and hepatitis B vaccines.
[187] Moskowitz, Richard MD. *Vaccines: A Reappraisal*. New York: Skyhorse Publishing, 2017, p. 127-129.
[188] Wakefield AJ, et al. Ileal Lymphoid-Nodular Hyperplasia, Non-Specific Colitis, and Pervasive Development Disorder in Children. *Lancet*, 1998; 351(673), Retracted.
[189] Ibid.
[190] Ibid.
[191] Moskowitz, Richard MD. *Vaccines: A Reappraisal*. New York: Skyhorse Publishing, 2017, p. 91.
[192] Ibid, p. 93.
[193] Ibid, p. 92.

invalidated his original study, and his findings have even been confirmed by multiple other studies.[194, 195, 196, 197]

Though a number of papers were subsequently published suggesting that there was no link between the MMR and autism, the CDC's main investigation on the subject[198] has been implicated in scientific fraud on a large scale. This came to light in 2014,[199] ten years after the original paper was published, when William Thompson, the paper's lead scientist and fourth author, came forward with information about the data manipulation. The removal of half the subjects from the original study effectively eliminated a statistically significant link between the MMR and an increased incidence of autism in African Americans, and an even higher incidence in African American males.[200] The link was even more significant during the time period recommended on the CDC's vaccination schedule (15-18 months). Thompson claimed that the CDC had deviated from its original analysis plan, omitted data, reformatted data to diminish statistical significance, destroyed documents, and obstructed justice.[201] While the CDC claims these allegations are false, Thompson would have little incentive to come forward with the information if it was indeed untrue, especially after observing the firestorm that attended Wakefield's data.

In 2013 the CDC released another study that evaluated exposure to vaccine antigens in children with and without autism, and found that there was no statistically significant difference.[202] This leads the organization to conclude on their website in no uncertain terms that "vaccine ingredients do not cause autism."[203] However, this argument completely ignores the fact that the most commonly proposed mechanism of vaccine-induced autism has nothing to do with the vaccine antigens; instead, it is thought to be mediated through the action of either a preservative in the vaccine (thimerosol, which contains mercury and is known to be neurotoxic[204]) or an adjuvant (any one of the forms of aluminum that are used in various vaccines, which are also known to be

---

[194] Ibid, p. 94 (Reference 29). This validation includes both his work on the relationship between gut abnormalities and the development of autism, which was the actual subject of the retracted paper, as well as confirmation of his suspicion that there may be a link with the MMR vaccine.
[195] Horvath K, et al. Gastrointestinal Abnormalities in Children with Autistic Disorder. *Journal of Pediatrics* 135:559, 1999; Ashwood P et al. Intestinal Lymphocyte Populations in Children with Regressive Autism. *Journal of Clinical Immunology*, 2003; 23(503).
[196] Singh V and Jensen R. Elevated Measles Antibodies in Children with Autism. *Pediatric Neurology* 2003, 28(1).
[197] Galiastatos P, et al. Autistic Enterocolitis: Fact or Fiction? *Canadian Journal of Gastroenterology* 2009; 23(95).
[198] DeStefano F, Bhasin TK, Thompson WW, Yeargin-Allsopp M, Boyle C. Age at First Measles-Mumps-Rubella Vaccination in Children With Autism and School-Matched Control Subjects: A Population-Based Study in Metropolitan Atlanta. *Pediatrics*, 2004 Feb; 113 (2): 259-266. https://doi.org/10.1542/peds.113.2.259
[199] Park A. Whistleblower Claims CDC Covered Up Data Showing Vaccine-Autism Link. *Time*, 28 Aug 2014. https://time.com/3208886/whistleblower-claims-cdc-covered-up-data-showing-vaccine-autism-link/ Accessed 29 Oct 2019.
[200] Bigtree A, Wakefield A, Tomney P. *Vaxxed: From Cover-Up to Catastrophe*. DVD. Burbank, CA: Cinema Libre, 2017.
[201] Ibid.
[202] DeStefano F, Price CS, Weintraub ES. Increasing Exposure to Antibody-Stimulating Proteins and Polysaccharides in Vaccines Is Not Associated with Risk of Autism. *Journal of Pediatrics*, 2013 Aug; 163(2): 561–567. https://doi.org/10.1016/j.jpeds.2013.02.001
[203] CDC. "Vaccines Do Not Cause Autism." https://www.cdc.gov/vaccinesafety/concerns/autism.html Accessed 29 Oct 2019.
[204] Geier DA, Sykes LK, Geier MR. A review of Thimerosal (Merthiolate) and its ethylmercury breakdown product: specific historical considerations regarding safety and effectiveness. *Journal of Toxicology and Environmental Health*, Part B, 2004; 10: 575–596. DOI: 10.1080/10937400701389875

neurotoxic[205]). The exposure to the vaccine antigen is generally not put forward as a possible trigger for autism, and so the study uses a misleading surrogate to dismiss concerns about vaccine safety.

Recent research by Dr. Theresa Deisher suggests yet another possible mechanism for the onset of vaccine-induced autism, one that has a particularly powerful explanatory power. Part of the difficulty of explaining autism is that a significant amount of evidence suggests that it is triggered by environmental factors. There is also a significant contrasting body of evidence suggesting that there is a genetic component to the disorder. A number of studies have shown a strong correlation between autism and *de novo* mutations.[206] These types of changes in the DNA arise "anew" in an individual and are not present in either parent. Hundreds of these mutations have been identified in nearly 1,000 individuals.[207] Yet there is no strong correlation between specific mutations and autism, and this is part of the mystery of the genetic component of the disease.

However, if Dr. Deisher is correct, this seemingly random assortment of *de novo* mutations has a very explicable biological mechanism, and this mechanism is linked directly to the presence of contaminant DNA in vaccines that use aborted fetal cells.* A 2013 study to determine effective methods for gene therapy demonstrated that doses as low as 1.9 ng/mL of foreign DNA were sufficient to induce successful gene modification in the recipient of the DNA.[208] This effectively inserts new DNA into the host, which results in *de novo* mutations. In vaccines made using aborted fetal cells, the DNA from the fetal cells cannot be purified out of the final vaccine preparation but remains as a contaminant. The DNA contamination can be as high as 175 ng per dose,[209] or nearly 350 ng/mL[210] - this is *over 180 times* the necessary threshold for the DNA to have an effect on the patient's genes. Since the contaminating DNA is human DNA, it is highly suitable for a role in genetic transformation of the patient because of its inherent similarity to the DNA of the individual

---

[205] Tomljenovic L, Shaw CA. Aluminum Vaccine Adjuvants: Are They Safe? *Curr Med Chem* 2011; 18(17): 2630-37.

[206] Sanders SJ, Murtha MT, State, MW. *De novo* mutations revealed by whole-exome sequencing are strongly associated with autism. *Nature*, 2012; 485: 237–241.

[207] Ibid.

* At the time of the writing of this paper, the following vaccines on the CDC's recommended schedule are made using aborted fetal cell lines: chickenpox (Varivax and Varilrix), hepatitis A (Vaqta, Havrix, Avaxim, Epaxal), hepatitis A & B (Twinrix), measles/mumps/rubella (MMR, Priorix), measles/rubella (MR Vax, Eolarix), mumps/rubella (Biavax II), rubella (Meruvax II), measles/mumps/rubella/chickenpox (ProQuad/MMR-V, Priorix Tetra), polio (Poliovax, DT PolAds, Polio Sabin), DTaP/polio/Hib (Pentacel, Quadracel, Infanrix-IPV-Hib), and a number of the candidates for the SARS-CoV-2 vaccine. For a more complete list of all vaccines that are derived from aborted fetal cells, visit the website of Children of God for Life at https://cogforlife.org/wp-content/uploads/vaccineListOrigFormat.pdf.

[208] Deisher T. "Open Letter to Legislators Regarding Fetal Cell DNA in Vaccines." 8 Apr 2019. Connecticut General Assembly, https://www.cga.ct.gov/kid/related/20190513_Informational%20Hearing%20on%20the%20State%27s%20Religious %20Exemption/Testimony/Testimony%20Theresa%20Deisher%20PhD.pdf Accessed 29 Oct 2019

This modification occurs through homologous recombination, where pieces of foreign DNA line up with similar sequences in the host's genome; proteins that are responsible for DNA modification then swap out the foreign DNA for the host DNA.

[209] Deisher T. "Open Letter to Legislators Regarding Fetal Cell DNA in Vaccines." 8 Apr 2019. Connecticut General Assembly, https://www.cga.ct.gov/kid/related/20190513_Informational%20Hearing%20on%20the%20State%27s%20Religious %20Exemption/Testimony/Testimony%20Theresa%20Deisher%20PhD.pdf Accessed 29 Oct 2019

[210] MMR dosage is 0.5 mL. CDC. "Administering the MMR Vaccine." https://www.cdc.gov/vaccines/vpd/mmr/hcp/administering-mmr.html Accessed 29 Oct 2019.

receiving the vaccine.[211]   This similarity also results in the DNA not being as effectively cleared from the patient's body as the antigenic components of the vaccine; thus, it can persist for long enough periods of time to make the possibility of genetic transformation worrisome.  Finally, identification of a retrovirus contaminant in the MMR vaccine,[212] which is able to aid the insertion of foreign DNA into a host's genome, makes this mechanism even more likely.

Finally, in confirmation of Dr. Wakefield's original suspicion that there might be a link between the MMR vaccine and autism, Dr. Deisher has identified a correlation between the removal of the MMR vaccine from the market in the United Kingdom, Norway and Sweden and a subsequent drop in autism rates.  When the vaccine was returned to market, the autism rates rose again.[213] This accidental experiment provided a clue to Dr. Deisher, who looked at change points in the autism incidence in the United States and determined if they were associated with an increase in the use of vaccines made in aborted fetal cells.  She discovered that at each point in time where there was a significant increase in autism rates there was also the introduction of one or more new vaccines that were made using aborted fetal cells.[214]  The effect observed was also dose dependent – the more fetal cell derived vaccines that are administered, the higher the increase in the rate of autism.[215]  This dose dependence lends a particular credibility to the MMR vaccine (and other aborted fetal vaccines) being causally associated with autism, and not just temporally correlated as is so often claimed.

Indeed, according to the Bradford Hill criteria – which have been used to determine causality in health outcomes and epidemics since the 1960s – there is an extremely strong case for a causal association between vaccines and autism.  Of the nine criteria that are considered, three of the most important are temporality, a biological gradient, and coherence:[216]

1. The temporal relationship between vaccination and the onset of autistic response is not debated even by the strongest vaccine proponents; and, interestingly, temporality is the only one of the nine criteria that is considered *absolutely essential for establishing causality*.
2. Dr. Deisher has shown that the relationship between vaccines and autism follows a biological gradient by demonstrating the dose-response that is observed when vaccination

---

[211] Deisher T. "Open Letter to Legislators Regarding Fetal Cell DNA in Vaccines." 8 Apr 2019.  Connecticut General Assembly,
https://www.cga.ct.gov/kid/related/20190513_Informational%20Hearing%20on%20the%20State%27s%20Religious%20Exemption/Testimony/Testimony%20Theresa%20Deisher%20PhD.pdf Accessed 29 Oct 2019
[212] Brown D. Unexpected protein found in measles-mumps vaccine. *The Washington Post.* 9 Dec 1995.
https://www.washingtonpost.com/archive/politics/1995/12/09/unexpected-protein-found-in-measles-mumps-vaccine/3af651bf-aa56-43db-8c95-b1aea019d650/ Accessed 18 May 2020.
[213] Deisher TA, Doan NV, Koyama K, Bwabye S. Epidemiologic and Molecular Relationship Between Vaccine Manufacture and Autism Spectrum Disorder Prevalence. *Issues Law Med.* 2015 Spring; 30(1): 47-70.
[214] Deisher, TA. "Worldwide Autism Epidemic & Human Fetal Manufactured Contaminated Vaccines." Presentation delivered at Autism One conference.  Uploaded to YouTube 10 Sept 2014.
https://www.youtube.com/watch?v=6Bc6WX33SuE Accessed 20 May 2019.
[215] Ibid.
[216] Yeats K and Alexander L, The University of North Carolina at Chapel Hill. Bradford Hill Criteria. In: Epidemiology: The Basic Science of Public Health. Coursera.
https://www.coursera.org/lecture/epidemiology/bradford-hill-criteria-qXlFt Accessed 2 April 2020.

with fetal-cell-derived vaccines is increased and there is a corresponding increase in autism rates.

3. Finally, the criteria of coherence, that states that new data should not oppose the current association,[217] is satisfied by the fact that there is a cluster of associated health effects that are all correlated with vaccination. Since autism has frequently been characterized as involving an autoimmune component,[218, 219] it fits coherently with other documented side effects of vaccination.

In addition, Dr. Deisher also provides a biologically plausible explanation for the effects observed, and supports both the mechanism and the association with experimental evidence, thus satisfying two more of the nine criteria. Thus the link between autism and vaccines easily satisfies the majority of the established criteria for epidemiological causality, and cannot be easily dismissed.

## *Shifting Susceptibility: How Vaccines Weaken a Population's Immunity*

Thus far, the dangers of vaccination to the individual have been discussed. However, vaccines also pose dangers to the vaccinated population as a whole. As this population is the subject of many "greater good" arguments in favor of mass vaccination, it is imperative to examine some of these problems in more detail.

One major issue for populations is that vaccines can cause a shift in the susceptible members of the population, which moves diseases into age-groups that normally would not contract them. Measles and chicken pox are well-known and convenient examples, but the general trends described can apply to nearly all of the childhood diseases that modern medicine attempts to prevent with vaccines.

While measles has been a relatively mild disease in the United States since sanitation and living conditions improved in the early half of the 20th century, it can be lethal in infants. Prior to the era of vaccination, infants of mothers who had contracted the disease were the recipients of a powerful form of passive immunity. Nursing infants received protective antibodies and immune cells[220] through the breast milk, and so did not generally contract the disease.[221] Vaccination, while it can prevent the mother from contracting a case of measles during her own childhood, impairs her ability to produce antibodies for the passive immunity of her infant[222] and prevents her from transmitting memory-activated T cells that would normally be passed through breast milk from a mother who had been naturally infected. Thus, infants born to vaccinated mothers are almost three

---

[217] Ibid.
The authors explicitly state that it is possible that conflicting information may be incorrect or highly biased, and we do see that with the CDC's study on autism and vaccines.
[218] Onore C, Careaga M, Ashwood P. The role of immune dysfunction in the pathophysiology of autism. *Brain Behav Immun*. 2012;26(3):383-392. doi:10.1016/j.bbi.2011.08.007
[219] Ashwood P, Krakowiak P, Hertz-Picciotto I, Hansen R, Pessah I, Van de Water J. Elevated plasma cytokines in autism spectrum disorders provide evidence of immune dysfunction and are associated with impaired behavioral outcome. *Brain Behav Immun*. 2011;25(1):40-45. doi:10.1016/j.bbi.2010.08.003
[220] Le Jan C. Cellular Components of Mammary Secretions and Neonatal Immunity: A Review. *Veterinary Research*, 1996; 27(4-5): 403-417.
[221] Miller, NZ. *Vaccines: Are They Really Safe and Effective?* Santa Fe: New Atlantean Press, 2018, p. 29-30.
[222] Papania M. Increased Susceptibility to Measles in Infants in the United States. *Pediatrics*, 1999 Nov; 1045(5), e59: 1-6.

times as likely to catch measles if they are exposed to it,* and the vulnerability to the disease is "shifted" towards this previously well-protected population – by the 1990s, more than 25% of all cases of measles were occurring in infants under 1 year of age.[223] This shift is a direct result of mass vaccination policy. Lack of infant immunity is an issue in the United States; while measles is no longer considered endemic in this country, measles outbreaks do occur and appear to be occurring with a cyclic pattern of increase in the number of cases.** Despite the hopes of vaccine proponents, we saw earlier that even 100% vaccination coverage can fail to achieve herd immunity sufficient to protect all infants from measles, due to both primary and secondary vaccine failure. Thus, the process of mass vaccination has created a new and potentially more deadly problem with this childhood illness by rendering infants vulnerable who were previously protected from infection.

This type of shift is not just the case for measles. Vaccination for many diseases simply does not provoke a sufficient immune response for a mother to provide the same passive immune protection to her baby as she would after a natural infection. This leaves her infant vulnerable, at a minimum, to measles, mumps, rubella, and chickenpox[224] (and possibly other diseases) at a time when the infant's immune system is insufficiently developed to handle these kinds of infectious agents. Natural infection, on the other hand, occurs at a time when the immune system is sufficiently

---

* The protection from maternal antibodies and immune cells is good, but not perfect. Only about 12% of infants born to naturally immune mothers contracted measles after being exposed to it; by comparison, approximately 33% of infants born to vaccinated mothers contracted measles after exposure to the virus.

[223] Miller, NZ. *Vaccines: Are They Really Safe and Effective?* Santa Fe: New Atlantean Press, 2018, p. 30.

** CDC. "Measles Cases and Outbreaks." Last updated 3 Oct 2019. https://www.cdc.gov/measles/cases-outbreaks.html. Accessed 29 Oct 2019.

     Note that the number of measles cases, while it has increased since 2010, is still extremely small compared to the overall population of the US. Approximately 0.00038% of the estimated population of the US contracted measles in 2019 (1250 cases as of Oct 3). Since 2010, there have been 3,208 cases of measles; the last verifiable death from measles occurred in 2003, when two infants died from measles (https://vaxopedia.org/2018/04/15/when-was-the-last-measles-death-in-the-united-states/). In contrast, using Dr. Sears' extremely conservative estimate of the rate of adverse reactions as 1 in 100,000 doses of vaccine, and the CDC's data concerning measles vaccination (approximately 116,000,000 doses of MMR and MMR-V administered between 2006 and 2016: https://www.hrsa.gov/sites/default/files/hrsa/vaccine-compensation/monthly-website-stats-2-01-18.pdf) the number of *severe* adverse reactions from the measles vaccine alone is estimated to be a minimum of 1,160 over an equivalent time period (but is likely to be closer to 11,600-116,000 given the insufficiency of the VAERS data). In the decade prior to the introduction of the measles vaccine, the CDC estimates 400-500 deaths from measles occurred each year (https://www.cdc.gov/measles/about/history.html), but they do not give actual statistics. This estimate is certainly inflated due to the fact that the clinical definition of measles was narrowed at the same time the vaccine was introduced (Humphries and Bystrianyk 2015, p. 371). Recent research has indicated that measles mortality is significantly reduced by proper nutrition (malnourished children are more than four times as likely to die from measles as healthy ones) and vitamin A supplementation (which can reduce measles mortality by up to 80%). Use of these two protocols would likely have reduced the death rate from measles to almost zero even without the vaccine (Humphries and Bystrianyk 2015, p. 340, 390-397). So, the population as a whole has traded a slight decrease in measles deaths for around 1,000-10,000 prolonged hospital stays, life-threatening illnesses, permanent disabilities, and deaths each year. As another note of comparison, while vaccine proponents like to use the rising incidence of measles to coerce more individuals into consenting to vaccination, more people in the US died from shark attacks in 2019 than have died from measles in the last fifteen years (https://people.com/human-interest/2019-us-shark-attacks-map/).

[224] Waaijenborg S, Hahné SJM, et al. Waning of Maternal Antibodies Against Measles, Mumps, Rubella, and Varicella in Communities With Contrasting Vaccination Coverage. *J Infect Dis*, 2013 Jul 1; 208(1): 10–16. https://doi.org/10.1093/infdis/jit143

mature to process these pathogens, and also when it is still undeveloped enough to be dramatically shaped by exposure to various childhood diseases.[225]

In other cases, we see a shift in susceptibility after vaccination that is not associated with declining maternal immunity. One primary example of this phenomenon is that vaccination for chickenpox has led to a substantial increase in the incidence of shingles.[226] (Both diseases are caused by the same virus, known as varicella-zoster.) Not only is the overall incidence of shingles on the rise, but the age of incidence is being driven lower by the mass vaccination program. Prior to vaccination, shingles was primarily a problem in adults over 60; but by 2004 this age group only accounted for 74% of shingles cases.[227] A New Zealand study further documented the decline in mean age of shingles cases, noting a decrease from 2007 to 2015 of 5.4 years of the average age of patients, as well as an overall increase in the number of patients from 71 to 195 per year.[228] In addition to this shift of susceptibility in the population at large, children are even contracting shingles from the chickenpox vaccine itself.[229]

What is particularly disconcerting about the data on shingles is that this shift in susceptibility was predicted *prior to the implementation of mass vaccination against chickenpox* and came as no surprise to clinical researchers.[230]

The primary proposed mechanism for the type of shift that we see with chickenpox and shingles is a loss of the protective effect of being exposed to wild-type disease after natural immunity has developed. It has been documented that caring for one's child through chickenpox can provide a protective effect against developing shingles as an adult.[231] As was mentioned earlier, we now know that natural immunity is not always permanent; it requires natural "boosting" from the circulation of the disease in the wild. Mass vaccination against chickenpox has effectively eliminated this natural boosting process and leaves individuals susceptible to shingles infection at younger and younger ages. It can readily be postulated that a similar phenomenon may be contributing to the resurgence of other "vaccine-preventable" diseases.

## Trading One Disease for Another: Vaccine Resistant Strains

Shifting susceptibility is not the only way that vaccines have made populations more vulnerable to disease. An even more insidious problem is strain replacement: when vaccination against one strain or species of pathogen allows other strains or species to become more prevalent in humans.

---

[225] Diodati CJM. *Immunization: History, Ethics, Law and Health*. Ontario, CN: Integral Aspects Incorporated, 1999, p. 51.

[226] Miller NZ. *Miller's Review of Critical Vaccine Studies*. Santa Fe: New Atlantean Press, 2016. References 181, 185, 187-192.

[227] Patel MS, Gebremariam A, Davis MM. Herpes Zoster–Related Hospitalizations and Expenditures Before and After Introduction of the Varicella Vaccine in the United States. *Infection Control and Hospital Epidemiology*, 2008 Dec; 29(12): 1157-116. https://doi.org/10.1086/591975

[228] Davies EC, Langston DP, Chodosh J. Herpes zoster opthalmicus: declining age at presentation. *Br J Ophthalmol*. 2016; 100: 312-314. doi:10.1136/bjophthalmol-2015-307157

[229] Miller NZ. *Miller's Review of Critical Vaccine Studies*. Santa Fe: New Atlantean Press, 2016. References 197-198.

[230] Ibid, References 193-194.

[231] Thomas SL, Wheeler JG, Hall AJ. Contacts with varicella or with children and protection against herpes zoster in adults: a case-control study. *Lancet* 2002 Aug 31; 360(9334): 678-82.

In some cases, the replacements cause even worse disease symptoms than the pathogens against which the vaccines are given.

It has been said that nature abhors a vacuum. In the complex interactions in the environment (and even in our bodies) involving bacteria, viruses, fungi, and other microorganisms, the niche created by eliminating one species or strain will quickly be filled by other opportunistic organisms. This is one reason why it is detrimental to overuse antibiotics; these drugs eliminate both pathogenic and helpful bacteria, and in some cases leave a void in the body's microbiome by killing off too many of the helpful type. Then species that are normally kept in check by competition can move into areas of the body they do not normally colonize and alter the microbial balance in the body overall. This can drive the development of disease in the body in ways that are still not well understood.

Antibiotic resistance is a rising problem in medicine of which everyone is aware. A similar, but less publicized scenario can be driven by the selective reduction of particular strains of pathogens through vaccination programs.[232] Some of the resurgence that has been observed among so-called vaccine preventable diseases is due to the rise of new strains or serotypes* of the particular pathogen. This has been documented for a number of specific vaccines. The pneumococcal and Hib vaccines protect against only a few serotypes of their respective pathogens, and other serotypes are gradually becoming more prevalent in the population.[233] This has led to overall higher rates of secondary vaccine failure with both of these vaccines. The same phenomenon is beginning to be observed with HPV vaccines as well.[234]

Pertussis (whooping cough) cases have increased substantially for several years despite good vaccination coverage, partly due to the increase of *Bordetella parapertussis* infections. *B. parapertussis* is normally at a very low circulation level in the environment when *Bordetalla pertussis* (the pathogen that normally causes whooping cough) is present in the population, but its prevalence has increased substantially since mass vaccination against *B. pertussis* began. *B. parapertussis* caused up to 16.5% of cases of whooping cough by 2012[235] and was also causing diseases in much younger children than *B. pertussis* (a mean age of 3.8 years vs. 15.6 years).[236] There are also substantial problems with *B. pertussis* strains that have emerged that have modified toxin proteins; these are not strains against which there is effective protection by vaccination.[237] Overall, these strain and species replacements may have reduced the pertussis vaccine efficacy to as low as 40%, an efficacy far below that needed to accomplish herd immunity in the population.[238]

---

[232] See Miller NZ. *Miller's Review of Critical Vaccine Studies*. Santa Fe: New Atlantean Press, 2016. References 116-126.

* A serotype is the technical term for a distinctive strain of a pathogen that can be distinguished in a test of the blood serum.

[233] Moskowitz R. *Vaccines: A Reappraisal*. New York: Skyhorse Publishing, 2017, p. 22-23.

[234] Fischer S, Bettstetter M, Becher A, et al. Shift in prevalence of HPV types in cervical cytology specimens in the era of HPV vaccination. *Oncology Letters*, 2016 Jul; 12(1). https://doi.org/10.3892/ol.2016.4668

[235] Cherry, JD. Why do pertussis vaccines fail? *Pediatrics*, 2012 May 1; 129(5): 968-70.

[236] Patel R. *Bordetella pertussis* and *Bordetella parapertussis*. Mayo Clinic Laboratories. 1 Oct 2018. https://news.mayocliniclabs.com/2018/10/01/bordetella-pertussis-and-bordetella-parapertussis/ Accessed 19 May 2020.

[237] See Miller NZ. *Miller's Review of Critical Vaccine Studies*. Santa Fe: New Atlantean Press, 2016. References 91-104.

[238] Cherry, JD. Why do pertussis vaccines fail? *Pediatrics*, 2012 May 1; 129(5): 968-70.

Yet another vaccine that is causing strain replacement is the HPV vaccine, which targets between two and nine strains of the virus (at the time of the writing of this paper, 150 different strains of HPV have been identified, though only some types cause serious pathology[239]). Gardasil®, the first vaccine for HPV, was initially fast-tracked through development because of the claim that it would help prevent cases of cervical cancer. When the vaccine was initially developed, HPV strains 16 and 18 accounted for most of the cases of cervical cancer in the target population.[240] However, recent studies have indicated a rise in other strains of HPV (particularly 53, 56, and 66) against which the current vaccines do not protect. HPV strains 53 and 66 are now known to be carcinogenic, as are strains 26, 67, 68, 70, 73 and 82 (which are not included in the vaccine's coverage either).[241] Thus, while the vaccine may result in an overall reduction in the HPV strains for which it is formulated, it will likely not result in any improvement in the rate of cervical cancer caused by HPV. This raises the issue of significant ethical problems with the way that the HPV vaccine was marketed as a cancer preventative, which will be more fully addressed in a subsequent section.

Vaccine-induced strain replacement phenomena spells trouble for the population as a whole. By reducing the circulation of one type of disease, vaccination can cause populations that are naïve (or previously unexposed) to the replacement pathogen to have higher rates of disease cases and also of mortality. It is possible, even likely, that there will be higher rates of death for these replacement strains than were observed for the original strains in the pre-vaccination era.

*Trading One Disease for Another: Cancer Rates on the Rise*

Another serious population-level problem associated with vaccines is increases in cancer rates that have occurred alongside the implementation of mass vaccination. Natural infections appear to prime the immune system in a way that makes it harder for cancer cells to take root in the body, and so provide a protective effect against many cancers that is not provided by vaccination. There is such an abundance of research in this area that it would be impossible to cover it all in the scope of this work, but a sampling of the findings is summarized in the following list:[242]

- Natural infection with mumps likely protects against ovarian cancer in women, and measles, rubella, and chickenpox may have similar protective effects.[243, 244, 245]

---

[239] NYU Langone Health. "Types of Human Papillomavirus." https://nyulangone.org/conditions/human-papillomavirus-in-adults/types Accessed 30 Oct 2019.

[240] Fischer S, Bettstetter M, Becher A, et al. Shift in prevalence of HPV types in cervical cytology specimens in the era of HPV vaccination. *Oncology Letters*, 2016 Jul; 12(1). https://doi.org/10.3892/ol.2016.4668

[241] Ibid.

[242] *See:* Miller NZ. *Miller's Review of Critical Vaccine Studies.* Santa Fe: New Atlantean Press, 2016. References 304-339.

[243] Newhouse ML, Pearson RM, et al. A case control study of carcinoma of the ovary. *Br J Prev Soc Med* 1977 Sep; 31(3): 148-53.

[244] Cramer DW, Vitonis AF, et al. Mumps and ovarian cancer: modern interpretation of an historic associate. *Cancer Causes Control* 2010 Aug; 21(8): 1193-1201.

[245] West RO. Epidemiologic study of malignancies of the ovaries. *Cancer* 1966; 19: 1001-17.

- The likelihood of malignant melanoma may be reduced by infection with chickenpox, influenza, measles, or mumps.[246, 247]
- Chickenpox and influenza infections are associated with a reduced risk of brain tumors.[248]
- Contracting measles, mumps, or rubella appears to be protective against non-Hodgkin's lymphomas.[249]
- The risk of developing Hodgkin's lymphoma is reduced by pertussis, measles, mumps, chickenpox, and influenza infections in childhood.[250, 251]
- Children who experienced diseases that caused fevers are protected against multiple cancers in adulthood, and the more frequent these diseases are contracted the less likely the children are to develop cancer.[252, 253]
- Early exposure to infections seems to be particularly protective against leukemia.[254, 255]

In addition to these specific examples, researchers have noticed a correlation between the reduction of infectious disease in modern times and the rise of cancer incidence.[256] This may be due to the fact that the body is able to destroy cancer cells during an immune response to an infectious disease.[257] Cancer cells display distinctive markers that allow them to be targeted and eliminated by immune cells, and if the immune system is properly primed through natural infection, this process appears to be more efficient. In addition, other studies have shown that exposure to infections in childhood is part of the process of developing a mature immune system, and that earlier exposures can significantly reduce the risk of some types of cancer.[258]

An even more remarkable find is that the measles virus itself has been shown to reverse the course of some types of cancer,[259] and is being explored as a possible therapeutic agent in cancer

[246] Kolmel KF, Gefeller O, et al. Febrile infections and malignant melanoma: results of a case-control study. *Melanoma Res* 1992; 2(3): 207-11.

[247] Kolmel KF, Pfahlberg A, et al. Infections and melanoma risk: results of a multicentre EORTC case-control study. European Organization for Research and Treatment of Cancer. *Melanoma Red* 1999; 9(5): 511-19.

[248] Schlehofer B, Blettner M, et al. Role of medical history in brain tumour development. Results from the international adult brain tumour study. *Int J Cancer* 1999 Jul 19; 82(2): 155-60.

[249] Rudant J, Orsi L, et al. Childhood Hodgkin's lymphoma, non-Hodgkin's lymphoma and factors related to the immune system: the Escale Study (SFCE). *Int J Cancer* 2011 Nov 1; 129(9): 2236-47.

[250] Ibid.

[251] Alexander FE, Jarrett RF, et al. Risk factors for Hodgkin's disease by Epstein-Barr virus (EBV) status: prior infection by EBV and other agents. *Br J Cancer* 2000 Mar; 82(5): 1117-21.

[252] Hoption Can SA, van Netten JP, et al. Acute infections as a means of cancer prevention: opposing effects to chronic infections? *Cancer Detect Prev* 2006; 30(1): 83-93.

[253] Mastrangelo G, Fadda E, Milan G. Cancer increased after a reduction of infections in the first half of this century in Italy: etiologic and preventive implications. *Eur J Epidemiol* 1998 Dec; 14(8): 749-54.

[254] van Steensel-Moll HA, Valkenburg HA, et al. Childhood leukemia and infectious diseases in the first year of life: a register-based case-control study. *Am J Epidemiol* 1986 Oct; 124(4): 590-94.

[255] Petridou E, Kassimos D, et al. Age of exposure to infections and risk of childhood leukaemia. *BMJ* 1993 Sep 25; 307: 774.

[256] Mastrangelo G, Fadda E, Milan G. Cancer increased after a reduction of infections in the first half of this century in Italy: etiologic and preventive implications. *Eur J Epidemiol* 1998 Dec; 14(8): 749-54.

[257] Ibid.

[258] Chang ET, Zheng T, et al. Childhood social environment and Hodgkin's lymphoma: new findings from a population-based case-control study. *Cancer Epidemiol Biomarkes Prev* 2004 Aug; 13(8): 1361-70.

[259] Wilson J, Hudson W. "Measles virus used to put woman's cancer into remisson." CNN. 18 May 2014. https://www.cnn.com/2014/05/15/health/measles-cancer-remission/index.html Accessed 30 Oct 2019.

treatment.[260] Infection with the chickenpox virus has also been identified as a possible therapy for malignant glioma cancers.[261] Both of these therapies are likely to be less effective in individuals who have been vaccinated for the diseases in question, and will probably require immunosuppressive therapy to be administered simultaneously with the therapeutic use of the virus.[262] Though the authors of the paper did not mention this fact, any immunosuppressive drugs will greatly reduce the body's ability to respond well to the treatment since it is the activated immune system that is responsible for eliminating the cancer cells.

---

[260] Russell SJ, Peng KW. Measles virus for cancer therapy. *Curr Top Microbiol Immunol.* 2009; 330: 213–241.
[261] Leska H, Hasse R, et al. Varicella zoster virus infection of malignant glioma cell cultures: a new candidate for oncolytic virotherapy? *Anticancer Res* 2012 Apr; 32(4): 1137-44.
[262] Russell SJ, Peng KW. Measles virus for cancer therapy. *Curr Top Microbiol Immunol.* 2009; 330: 213–241.

# The Morality of Vaccination

*I assert that it is beyond the functions of law*
*to dictate a medical procedure, or enforce any scientific theory.*
*-- Emeritus Professor F. W. Newman[263]*

Throughout this work, there have been a number of allusions to specific ethical and moral issues that are at stake when decisions must be made about how vaccines are manufactured, marketed, and administered. This chapter will address the issues of appropriate consideration for the safety of whole populations (particularly the argument that the achievement and maintenance of herd immunity is of greater ethical and moral concern than an individual's choice to vaccinate or not vaccinate) as well as addressing concerns for the safety of the individual (particularly the grave moral concerns regarding aborted fetal vaccines, but also concerns regarding the possibility of infertility and the administration of vaccines in ways that are unreasonable). At the end of the chapter, the ethical issues of vaccine manufacturing and the reporting of adverse events will also be canvassed.

## The Ethics of Herd Immunity

One of the most common arguments for mandatory vaccination is that it is necessary for the maintenance of herd immunity. Herd immunity becomes an ethical issue because it is thought to protect the most vulnerable members of society and those who often cannot receive a vaccine themselves: immunocompromised individuals, pregnant mothers, and infants. Vaccine proponents often insist that individual choice regarding vaccinations should be overruled because the only way to maintain the safety of vulnerable individuals in the face of infectious disease is to ensure that a sufficient number of individuals are vaccinated.[264] Even the argument put forward by the Pontifical Academy for Life (PAL) about the possibility of aborted vaccines being ethically permissible ultimately rests on the foundation of herd immunity, specifically through the protection of susceptible populations (pregnant women) by the vaccination of other populations (children).[265] The specific argument from the PAL will be addressed in the next section on aborted fetal vaccines. First, it is important to establish an understanding of the nature of herd immunity, and whether or not it is a reasonable argument for driving vaccination policy.

Mary Holland and Chase Zachary argue that herd immunity is based on five "core" assumptions that are not upheld in real epidemiological situations[266]:

1. population homogeneity (in terms of race, social/economic status, and genetics);
2. well-mixing of the population (each individual having an identical chance of being exposed to an infected person);

---

[263] As quoted in Humphries S and Bystrianyk R. *Dissolving Illusions*. Printed by author. 2015, p. 141.
[264] NOVA. *Vaccines: Calling the Shots*, 2014. DVD. Boston: PBS.
[265] "Moral Reflections on Vaccines Prepared from Cells Derived from Aborted Human Foetuses," Potifica Academia Pro Vita, June 9, 2005. https://www.ncbcenter.org/files/1714/3101/2478/vaticanresponse.pdf Accessed May 20 and August 13, 2019.
[266] Holland M, Zachary CE. Herd Immunity and Compulsory Childhood Vaccination: Does the Theory Justify the Law? *Oregon Law Review*, 2014; 93(1): 1-48.

3.  random vaccination of individuals (assuming that individuals with high risk for the disease are vaccinated at the same rates as individuals with low risk; the latter requires much more extensive vaccine coverage than targeting high-risk populations for vaccination);[*]
4.  perfect vaccine efficacy; and
5.  age uniformity in the population (assuming that individuals in all age groups have equal protection from vaccination, despite differing policies in vaccinating children vs. adults).

We have already discussed the case against perfect vaccine efficacy. While Holland and Zachary's paper in the *Oregon Law Review* has a fuller treatment of each objection they raise, ultimately the problem boils down to the fact that not all individuals are equally susceptible or equally likely to transmit the disease, so the vaccination of a certain random percentage of individuals does not eliminate the possibility of disease transmission. Instead, the authors argue that disease can be contained more effectively through elective vaccination, as well as arguing that disease containment is a much more attainable and helpful goal than the elusive eradication of disease.[♦]

A particular problem with the ethics of the herd immunity argument arises in light of vaccine failure rates that exceed the threshold for herd immunity. For example, as mentioned earlier, herd immunity against measles requires that a population be 95% immune; but the failure rate of the vaccine may be as high as 15%, exceeding the 5% non-immune threshold. In such cases, even with a 100% vaccination rate, there is no possible way to ensure herd immunity in a population. Even if the failure rate were 5% or lower, herd immunity still may be an unreachable goal because 100% vaccination is never attainable, as there are individuals in the population who cannot be vaccinated (per the CDC's list of definite contraindications).[267] Because of these factors, arguments based on a perceived greater good to society by enforcing mass vaccination are invalid – such a goal is simply unattainable in practice. Holland and Zachary go to some lengths to demonstrate the mathematics of this principle; it is sufficient for our purposes to understand its general application.

It could also be argued that the herd immunity argument put forward for mandatory mass vaccination is actually a much better argument for refraining from vaccinating for any new diseases altogether. When a disease passes through a population, it produces natural herd immunity, and this threshold is neither arbitrary nor unattainable, as it is with artificial induction of the immune response through vaccination. The immune system does not have the same failure rate as vaccines.

---

[*] Disease transmission dynamics differ in high and low risk populations. Holland and Zachary make the case that if a high-risk population requires 80% vaccine coverage to attain herd immunity, and this group was specifically targeted for vaccination, the total vaccine load on the population might be as low as 40%. However, if 80% of all individuals were randomly vaccinated this would not necessarily achieve herd immunity in the high-risk population, and the disease might still spread among susceptible individuals despite high rates of national vaccination.

[♦] Disease eradication was defined by A. Hinman as "permanent reduction to zero of the worldwide incidence of infection caused by a specific agent as a result of deliberate efforts" at which point "intervention is no longer needed." Such a process involves a huge effort to develop, manufacture, and distribute vaccines, as well as efficient tracking of cases of the disease around the globe. If vaccines cannot generate herd immunity, as we have seen that they cannot, they certainly cannot bring about disease eradication. (Holland & Zachary, 2014)

[267] CDC. Who should not get vaccinated? 2 Apr 2020. https://www.cdc.gov/vaccines/vpd/should-not-vacc.html Accessed 19 Sept 2020.

*Vaccines and Abortion*

The Pontifical Academy for Life (PAL) released a statement in 2005 regarding the morality of using vaccines containing aborted fetal cells. The document gave discerning parents sufficient reason to either reject or submit to the vaccine[268] and so the statement did not provide definite guidance to concerned Catholics. Commentators on online Catholic news websites further obfuscate the situation by misrepresenting the nuanced statements of the bishops regarding the gravity of these vaccines,[269] and by representing web pages with unidentified authors[270] as carrying equal authority to a formal letter by the PAL. Neither the formal letter nor the website is, in point of fact, dogmatically binding. Both statements are problematic in light of sound biological science as well as traditional Catholic moral teaching and philosophical principles. I will unpack this claim, as it raises serious concerns.

The following paragraph from the 2005 statement by the PAL is used by some to claim that the Vatican has granted permission for the use of aborted fetal vaccines because of the nature of the participation in the evil of abortion – which is considered, in this case, to be passive and remote – and because of the gravity of not vaccinating:

> As regards the diseases against which there are no alternative vaccines which are available and ethically acceptable, it is right to abstain from using these vaccines if it can be done without causing children, and indirectly the population as a whole, to undergo significant risks to their health. However, if the latter are exposed to considerable dangers to their health, vaccines with moral problems pertaining to them may also be used on a temporary basis. The moral reason is that the duty to avoid passive material cooperation is not obligatory if there is grave inconvenience. Moreover, we find, in such a case, *a proportional reason*, in order to accept the use of these vaccines in the presence of the danger of favouring the spread of the pathological agent, due to the lack of vaccination of children. This is particularly true in the case of vaccination against German measles.[271] [Emphasis in original]

Since the strongest example the PAL gives in favor of vaccination is rubella (German measles), it behooves us to take a closer look at this disease:

---

[268] "Moral Reflections on Vaccines Prepared from Cells Derived from Aborted Human Foetuses," Pontifica Academia Pro Vita, June 9, 2005. https://www.ncbcenter.org/files/1714/3101/2478/vaticanresponse.pdf Accessed May 20 and August 13, 2019.

[269] "What Does the Catholic Church Teach about Vaccines," Catholic News Agency, May 6, 2019. https://www.catholicnewsagency.com/news/what-does-the-catholic-church-teach-about-vaccines-75223 Accessed May 20, 2019.

[270] "Note on Italian vaccine issue," Pontifical Academy for Life, July 31, 2017. http://www.academyforlife.va/content/pav/en/the-academy/activity-academy/note-vaccini.html Accessed May 20, 2019.

[271] "Moral Reflections on Vaccines Prepared from Cells Derived from Aborted Human Foetuses," Potifica Academia Pro Vita, June 9, 2005. https://www.ncbcenter.org/files/1714/3101/2478/vaticanresponse.pdf , accessed May 20 and August 13, 2019.

- Rubella is generally a mild disease in children and does not generally require a trip to the family doctor.[272]
- It is so mild that it may be missed altogether in up to half of patients who contract the illness.[273]
- The disease is not dangerous to infants or children, but may cause arthritis if contracted by adults. [274]
- The primary danger posed by the disease occurs if it is contracted by a pregnant woman, particularly in the first twelve weeks of pregnancy.[275]
- If the infant *in utero* contracts rubella from the mother, miscarriage or stillbirth may result. Children that survive the infection often have congenital rubella syndrome (CRS), which may manifest as blindness, deafness, heart defects, and a host of other physiological issues.[276]

Congenital rubella syndrome is indeed a serious medical condition, and it would be ideal if it could be treated or prevented altogether. But the ideal of disease eradication is not the question of immediate concern. Rather, it is a more practical question: does childhood vaccination against rubella protect effectively against the possibility of pregnant women contracting rubella and protect their children from developing from CRS? It appears to do no such thing. Instead, childhood vaccination against rubella has pushed the susceptibility to the disease into an older age bracket, much as we saw with chickenpox/shingles in our last section. Since the licensing of the rubella vaccine in 1969, women of childbearing age are *more* likely to contract the disease than they were prior to the vaccine era, and the first few years after vaccine introduction were marked by a spike in the number of cases of CRS.[277] We have already discussed CRS occurring in infants whose mothers had high antibody titers, and were thus thought to be fully immune to contracting rubella. In addition to this, it has been noted that mothers who have been *repeatedly* vaccinated for rubella have still given birth to infants affected by CRS.[278] And while it is true that total numbers of CRS cases per year began to decline in the 1980s, this was not until over a decade after the vaccine's introduction, and has been attributed as much or more to declining fertility rates and elective abortions after rubella exposure than to protection from CRS via vaccination.[279, 280]

Another ethical concern must be addressed here. Since children are not the population that is actually susceptible to damage from rubella, we have here a clear case of advocating the induction of herd immunity in one population to protect a different, susceptible population. Effective herd immunity for protection of women of childbearing age against rubella is approximately 80-85%.

[272] Miller, NZ. *Vaccines: Are They Really Safe and Effective?* Santa Fe: New Atlantean Press, 2018, p. 33. *See also:* notes 166 and 167 from the same book.
[273] Thomas P and Margulis J. *The Vaccine-Friendly Plan.* New York: Ballantine Books, 2016, p. 186-187.
[274] Sears RW. *The Vaccine Book.* New York: Little, Brown and Company, 2011, p. 83
[275] CDC. Pregnancy and Rubella. 15 Sept 2017. https://www.cdc.gov/rubella/pregnancy.html Accessed 21 Apr 2020.
[276] Ibid.
[277] Diodati CJM. *Immunization: History, Ethics, Law and Health.* Ontario, CN: Integral Aspects Incorporated, 1999, p. 18.
[278] Ibid, p. 32.
[279] Ibid, p. 19.
[280] Ravitz J. Before Zika: The virus that helped legalize abortion in the US. *CNN*, 11 Aug 2016. https://www.cnn.com/2016/08/09/health/rubella-abortion-zika/index.html. Accessed 21 April 2020.

However, naturally occurring rubella infection, which is harmless in the vast majority of the population, already produced at least 80% herd immunity before the induction of vaccination.[281] As evidenced by the spike in CRS immediately following vaccination, it is likely that the natural herd immunity had already provided better protection for vulnerable infants *in utero* than the vaccine program could have, and it presented significantly less risk for the children who are being vaccinated. Thus, we can reasonably conclude, from a validated medical viewpoint, that there is *not* a "proportional reason" to accept the use of aborted fetal vaccines. Indeed, rubella vaccination instead *increases* the overall risk of "considerable danger to health" that the PAL document states we have permission to avoid.

Let us turn now to the second, and more important, piece of the puzzle: the question of whether the use of aborted-fetal-cell derived vaccines could be in accord with Catholic moral principles under any circumstances. Fr. Phil Wolfe[282] and Fr. Michael Copenhagen[283] have both written excellent explanations of the specific moral problems involved in the use of aborted fetal vaccines. Their arguments are briefly summarized in the following paragraphs.

In more than one instance, an argument has been made that the proximity of the person being vaccinated is sufficiently remote from the evil of the abortion (whence the material used in the vaccine was obtained) to justify the liceity of receiving the vaccine.[284] Fr. Michael Copenhagen points out that these arguments are insufficient, however, as they ignore the participation in actual sin by individuals who use the aborted remains:

> [A]n assessment of cooperation with evil in terms of distance from the original abortion is a necessary but ultimately insufficient criterion because there is another distinct and more immediate category of sin involved. [...] The recipient is an immediate participant in the commission of *continuous theft of human remains obtained through deliberate killing*, their *desecration through exploitation and trafficking*, as well as *ultimate omission to respectfully bury them*. While the original killing establishes the illicit character of using the remains, their possession and use becomes a distinct evil in itself, the circumstances of which do not cease as a form of theft, desecration, exploitation, and refusal to bury, regardless of the consumer's distance in time from the abortion, or the number of cell divisions, or the merely sub-cellular fragmentary inclusion of the child's DNA and protein in the final dose.[285] [Emphasis added]

Fr. Wolfe explains that use of aborted fetal vaccines is further in violation of the principle of the integral good – that is, the principle that in order for an act to be good, all of its parts must be

[281] Diodati CJM. *Immunization: History, Ethics, Law and Health.* Ontario, CN: Integral Aspects Incorporated, 1999, p.18-19.

[282] Wolfe P. The Morality of using Vaccines derived from Fetal Tissue Cultures: A Few Considerations. 07 May 2012. https://cogforlife.org/fr-phil-wolfe/ Accessed 20 May 2019.

[283] Copenhagen M. Restore Ye to Its Owners: on the immorality of receiving vaccines derived from abortion. 16 Oct 2019. https://cogforlife.org/wp-content/uploads/VaccineFrCopenhagen.pdf Accessed 6 Nov 2019.

[284] Wong A. The Ethics of HEK-293. Originally published in the National Catholic Bioethics Quarterly, 2006 Autumn; 6.3: 473–495. https://pdfs.semanticscholar.org/65a7/5696bb1e03a46cba9f0c976da2b50916dec2.pdf Accessed Apr 2011.

[285] Copenhagen M. Restore Ye to Its Owners: on the immorality of receiving vaccines derived from abortion. 16 Oct 2019. https://cogforlife.org/wp-content/uploads/VaccineFrCopenhagen.pdf Accessed 6 Nov 2019.

good.[286] This means that both the end (the desired goal) and the means to that end (the steps taken to secure the end) must *all* be good - or at least morally neutral - in order for the act to be good. If any one of these parts are evil, then the whole act is rendered evil. This principle is more commonly known as "the ends do not justify the means." While it can be reasonably argued that protecting one's children from the possibility of infectious disease is a morally good end, the means required to secure this end cannot be evil; if they are, the entire action is rendered evil. In the case of aborted fetal vaccines, the means required to reach the end of protecting the child's health are gravely evil. The means to the end of creating the vaccine involves using aborted fetal cells, which required the grave evil of abortion to be obtained.

It is important to establish exactly why such a use is evil, and why it cannot be argued that at least some good is coming out of an evil act by putting the cells to use in making medical discoveries. There are three important facets of explaining the nature of the evil involved: first, the use is evil because the vaccine would not exist except for the mortal sin that was committed; second, the use is evil because it constitutes possession in bad faith of something that was illicitly obtained (stolen); finally, the use is evil because it violates transcendent justice (the justice owed to God by human beings).

In justice, if one steals from another, one is obliged to at least return the stolen goods to the original owner, along with anything obtained through the stolen goods, and also to make up any additional loss suffered by the owner.[287] Strictly speaking, this manner of restitution is impossible in the case of the tissue of an aborted baby – but its impossibility does not excuse the researcher who goes on using the tissues for scientific discoveries. As Father Wolfe observes, "No power on Earth can give anyone the right to possess, purchase, or preserve tissue taken from a sacrificed baby."[288] Real restitution can – and should – be made by allowing the baby's tissues to die a natural death so that the evil is no longer being perpetuated. In other words, although restitution cannot be made in terms of giving the child its life back, the closest restitution possible is to properly bury the child. This "gives the body back to God" who is the only being who still has any rights over it[289] – thus it satisfies transcendent justice, which is violated by the continued use of the aborted fetal cells.

Moral theologian and PhD philosopher Fr. Chad Ripperger re-affirms this position, for he observes that because these vaccines are made from fetal tissue, insofar as the vaccine is a "fruit" of this fetal tissue, the vaccines and all of the vaccination materials must be buried.[290] The fetal tissue should have been buried in the first place, so whatever the tissue is illicitly used to create must be treated like the fetal tissue itself. In other words, since the fetal tissue should have been buried, if it is used to make the vaccine, the vaccine is to be buried and cannot be used for vaccinations.[291] Use of these vaccines does not then constitute only "remote" and "material" participation in

---

[286] Wolfe P. The Morality of using Vaccines derived from Fetal Tissue Cultures: A Few Considerations. 07 May 2012. https://cogforlife.org/fr-phil-wolfe/ Accessed 20 May 2019.

[287] Ibid.

[288] Ibid.

[289] Wolfe P. The Morality of using Vaccines derived from Fetal Tissue Cultures: A Few Considerations. 07 May 2012. https://cogforlife.org/fr-phil-wolfe/ Accessed 20 May 2019.

[290] Ripperger C. The Natural Law and Bioethics. 24 Jan 2014. https://www.youtube.com/watch?v=cCS34zDgTXQ&t=3892s&ab_channel=SensusFidelium Accessed 9 Sept 2020.

[291] Ibid.

something evil, but a much more direct participation in the use of immorally obtained fetal tissue. Thus, it is illicit for a Catholic to use something derived from these tissues – whether it be a vaccine or any other medical intervention – because this prolongs the time in which a present evil is being perpetuated.

Fr. Copenhagen further adds that this use of fetal-cell-derived vaccines is not a temporary solution – the acceptance and use of the aborted fetal vaccines only fuels the market for their continued use in medical research and contributes to the justification for expanding the use of aborted fetal cell lines.[292] As a researcher whose own scientific career was derailed by a refusal to participate in the use of these aborted remains, I can validate Father's supposition. There is an entire industry built around supporting the growth of aborted fetal cells in the laboratory, with special growth media, transfection reagents, analysis kits, and other laboratory paraphernalia all geared towards growing them under ideal conditions in the laboratory.[293] The more that these cells are used, and the more this research is documented in the literature and produces the "fruit" of marketable products, the more the evil will be perpetuated. Lest the reader dismiss the preceding argument as a mere supposition, it should be added here that new aborted fetal cell lines have been generated for laboratory use as recently as 2015. This was the Walvax2 cell line, which was developed by researchers in China to replicate the WI-38 and MRC-2 cell lines.[294] Due to all these factors, it is reasonable to assert that we have a moral obligation to *not* participate in this grave exploitation of innocent human beings.

While the PAL document seems to give permission to use the vaccines under certain circumstances without pain of sin, the permission to vaccinate with aborted-fetal-derived vaccines stands in direct contradiction to sound moral principles and it is difficult to see how this permission is justified. Additionally, as we have seen, the inconvenience of not vaccinating is not grave, and the risk to the individual exposed to the aborted fetal contaminants is grave indeed, further invalidating the arguments offered in the document.

### Infertility and Vaccination

There is another important pro-life issue that should be discussed in any treatise on vaccination: the possibility of infertility resulting from receiving certain vaccines. This is generally not a side effect that patients are warned about, and in some cases it appears to be an intended effect of the vaccine itself. Both situations raise serious ethical questions.

Recent research suggests that the human papillomavirus vaccine has the unintended side effect of significantly reducing fertility. A study collecting data on birth rates among females aged 25-29 in the United States showed a positive correlation between infertility and having received one or more doses of the HPV vaccine. Among the 8 million women who reported data on pregnancies,

---

[292] Copenhagen M. Restore Ye to Its Owners: on the immorality of receiving vaccines derived from abortion. 16 Oct 2019. https://cogforlife.org/wp-content/uploads/VaccineFrCopenhagen.pdf Accessed 6 Nov 2019.

[293] A quick search on Fisher Scientific for HEK 293 yields 15 products optimized for the use of this cell line and over 1,000 hits for documents supporting research questions concerning the cells: https://www.thermofisher.com/search/results?query=hek%20293&focusarea=Search%20All Accessed 19 May 2020.

[294] Vinnedge, D. Vaccines from Abortion – Time to Report the Truth! 20 May 2019. https://cogforlife.org/2019/05/20/vaccinetruth/ Accessed 27 May 2019.

60% of women who did not receive the HPV vaccine had been pregnant at least once, while only 35% of women who had received the vaccine had been pregnant. The study also reported that the chances of a woman becoming pregnant decreased with each additional dose of the vaccine.[295]

In addition to these statistics, case studies are emerging showing primary or premature ovarian failure (POF) associated with the HPV vaccine.[296,297] POF has been defined as "the onset of menopause before age 40" and it has been postulated that it can occur via an autoimmune mechanism.[298] Further study is needed to confirm whether this is the mechanism for the lowered incidence of pregnancy reported among women who have received the vaccine, but it is a reasonable biological candidate. It also suggests that HPV-vaccine-induced infertility is likely to be permanent.

While infertility after HPV-vaccine may be an unintended side effect, there are other vaccines that are intended to disrupt women's fertility. These vaccines are generally administered in Third World countries and their sterilizing effect is not disclosed. A notable recent case occurred in Kenya, when tetanus vaccines administered during a 2014 campaign were found to contain sterilizing agents.[299] These vaccines were developed and disseminated by the World Health Organization (WHO), which has been researching methods to achieve birth control through vaccines since the mid-1970s.[300] What is particularly troubling in this instance is that the vaccines were administered and primarily targeted to women of childbearing age without providing them with informed consent of the contraceptive nature of the vaccine vials. While WHO has disputed this charge, it remains a fact that vials of the vaccine that were obtained by Kenyan researchers tested positive for human chorionic gonadotropin (hCG), a chemical that causes miscarriages and infertility when administered simultaneously with the tetanus toxoid.[301] This is not the first time

---

[295] DeLong, Gayle. A lowered probability of pregnancy in females in the USA ages 25-29 who received a human papillomavirus injection. *Journal of Toxicology and Environmental Health,* 2018; 81(14): 661-674.

It should be noted that this paper was retracted in December of 2019, with the following reason given by the journal: "All of the post-publication reports we received described serious flaws in the statistical analysis and interpretation of the data in this paper, and we have therefore taken the decision to retract it." However, the author has written a rebuttal of the retraction, which is published here: https://childrenshealthdefense.org/news/hpv-article-withdrawn-without-detailed-explanation-by-journal-of-toxicology-and-environmental-health/. No detailed statistical analysis of the original paper was published by the journal or shared with the author, and the original analysis was not disputed by the peer-reviewers (nor by one of the secondary reviewers who looked at the paper prior to its retraction). While it is possible that there are some confounding factors in the original analysis – including the use of birth control or a lowered rate of pregnancy among college-educated females – the author did express in the original paper that the conclusions were limited and the results merited further investigation. Given the case study data that is available on HPV and infertility, her conclusions do not seem unreasonable.

[296] Little and Ward. Adolescent Premature Ovarian Insufficiency Following Human Papillomavirus Vaccination. *Journal of Investigative Medicine High Impact Case Reports*, 2014 Oct-Dec: 1-12. DOI: 10.1177/2324709614556129

[297] Colafrancesco, et al. Human Papillomavirus Vaccine and Primary Ovarian Failure: Another Facet of the Autoimmune/Inflammatory Syndrome Induced by Adjuvants. *American Journal of Reproductive Immunology*, 2013. DOI: 10.1111/aji.12151

[298] DeLong, Gayle. A lowered probability of pregnancy in females in the USA ages 25-29 who received a human papillomavirus injection. *Journal of Toxicology and Environmental Health,* 2018; 81(14): 661-674.

[299] Oller JW, et al. HCG Found in WHO Tetanus Vaccine in Kenya Raises Concern in the Developing World. *Open Access Library Journal*, 2017, Vol 4, e3937.

[300] Ibid, *see also:* notes 4-24 in the same article.

[301] Ibid. Also, personal communication with author Wahome Ngare.

that such a vaccination campaign has been pushed on an unsuspecting populace: similar attempts have been made in Mexico, Nicaragua, and the Philippines.[302]

## Unnecessary Administration

It could be argued that vaccine administration is generally unnecessary; but even if one grants that vaccines ought to be administered, there are a number of questionable practices regarding the number and timing of vaccinations. Booster shots of the MMR, for example, are not given to increase the length of immunity to measles, mumps, or rubella, but to attempt to induce an antibody response in children who experienced primary vaccine failure with the first vaccine.[303] Dr. Robert Sears estimates that this failure occurs in around 5% of children (though as we have seen in a prior section, it may be up to 15% of children). Regardless of whose statistics are correct, the vast majority of children who receive a second MMR shot (85-95%) are receiving an absolutely unnecessary dose of the vaccine, along with all its attendant risks; and it is not standard practice to screen children for protective antibody titers prior to administering these boosters, but simply to administer them indiscriminately to all individuals.

The hepatitis B (HepB) and HPV vaccines also raise ethical questions about necessity and timing of administration. The HepB vaccine is given to most infants within days of birth. But the disease against which the vaccine protects is primarily transmitted through intravenous drug use or having multiple sexual partners. Newborns are not at risk for either of these modes of transmission. There is, however, a substantial risk of transmission from an infected mother to an infant during delivery; but there are immunosuppressive drugs that reduce the risk of transmission almost to zero.[304] While children are still somewhat likely to contract the disease from an infected parent (about a 1 in 3 chance), the incidence of hepatitis B in the general population is quite low (at around 1%).[305] This means that roughly 99% of infants who receive this vaccine are not at risk for the disease at the time they are being vaccinated; they are also are at a higher risk for secondary vaccine failure if they move into a high-risk population as teenagers or young adults.

HPV vaccines, as they are protective against another sexually transmitted disease, are often seen by parents as unnecessary, and even as encouraging children in promiscuity. These vaccines are recommended for teens from 11-18 years of age, but are approved for children as young as nine, and adults up to 26 years of age.[306, 307] While HPV is a common infection among sexually active individuals, the vaccine only protects against nine strains of the virus (at most) and may actually lead individuals to run a greater risk of catching the other strains if they engage in risky sexual behavior. This is a common occurrence among young people when they think they are "protected" by interventions. In addition to these concerns, there are questions about the safety and efficacy of HPV vaccines, particularly Merck's Gardasil®. Gardasil® has one of the highest frequencies of

---

[302] Ibid.

[303] Sears RW. *The Vaccine Book.* New York: Little, Brown and Company, 2011, p. 93.

[304] Ibid, p. 47-53.

[305] Ibid, p. 47-51.

[306] Ibid, p. 154.

[307] CDC. Recommended Child and Adolescent Immunization Schedule for ages 18 years or younger, United States, 2020. 3 Feb 2020. https://www.cdc.gov/vaccines/schedules/hcp/imz/child-adolescent.html#note-hpv Accessed 20 April 2020

adverse reactions reported to the Vaccine Adverse Event Reporting System (VAERS)[308] and is associated with neurological damage, autoimmune onset, and even death. This is a risky set of trade-offs to take on for a disease which is easily preventable by behavior modification (which has no life-threatening side effects).

In addition, the fact that the HPV vaccine is marketed as an antidote to cervical cancer at all stretches the boundaries of credibility. It has been documented that regular Pap testing has decreased deaths from cervical cancer by 70%.[309] The implementation of this type of screening in countries where death rates are still high would likely have a far more positive impact than any vaccination campaign. Conversely, the implementation of mass vaccination in the US was unlikely to affect the death rate significantly even if the vaccine were protective against cancer, due to the already high incidence of Pap testing in the US. However, there is no evidence to suggest that the vaccine has any positive impact on the incidence of cervical cancer at all. Since this type of cancer can take decades to develop, and the original safety trial follow-ups for Merck's HPV vaccine Gardasil® lasted only five years, there was no possible way to detect any impact on cervical cancer rates, favorable or unfavorable. Instead, Merck tracked pre-cancerous lesions as a surrogate endpoint.[310] Normally, many of these lesions resolve without any treatment and do not develop into cancer, [311] which renders them a particularly misleading indicator of the vaccine's efficacy.

While it is reasonable to conclude, based on our prior discussion of safety and vaccines, that all vaccine administration is unnecessary, it is troubling that the medical establishment is so comfortable administering them in ways that would be unnecessary even if vaccines were wholly safe and effective.

### Ethical Issues in Vaccine Manufacturing

The method of conducting safety trials for vaccines is another area that is rife with ethical questions. The withholding of pharmaceutical trial data, biased towards only publishing positive results, is a ubiquitous problem in medicine. Sometimes trials that show little or no benefit from a drug are never published at all. In other cases, trials are stopped early or are too short to begin with, testing is done against a "placebo" that does not help the researchers identify possible adverse reactions to the drug under study, the main outcome is changed during or after the trial, or there are insufficient participants to identify anything except extremely common side effects.[312] Vaccines are no exception to this unfortunate trend.

Dr. Robert Sears identifies four major problems in vaccine safety studies that have not been adequately addressed:[313]

---

[308] Tomljenovic L and Shaw CA. Too Fast or Not Too Fast: The FDA's Approval of Merck's HPV Vaccine Gardasil. *Conflicts of Interest in the Practice of Medicine*, 2012 Fall: 673-681.
[309] Ibid.
[310] Ibid.
[311] Ostor AG. Natural History of Cervical Intraepithelial Neoplasia: A Critical Review. *Int J Gyn Path,* 1993; 12(2): 186-192.
[312] For a detailed study of this subject, see: Goldacre B. *Bad Pharma.* New York: Faber and Faber, 2012.
[313] Sears RW. *The Vaccine Book.* New York: Little, Brown and Company, 2011, p. 183-191.

1. Vaccines are not necessarily studied singly. Hib, pneumococcal, and polio vaccines, as well as one version of the DTaP vaccine, were tested only in combination with other vaccines. This makes it much more difficult to determine if there are adverse reactions to the newly developed vaccine. Any statistically significant difference in adverse reactions between the control group and the experimental group may be masked by reactions to other vaccines used in the study.

2. On the other hand, many vaccines are not studied in combination with the specific vaccines with which they are routinely administered. Some trials that conducted stand-alone studies of new vaccines include HPV, hepB, Tdap, chickenpox, and meningococcal vaccines, as well as an alternate version of the DTaP vaccine. These vaccines are routinely given with multiple other vaccines during clinical visits, but no testing has been done to determine if there is a synergistic effect between the specific vaccines that are simultaneously administered.

3. Vaccines are often studied in very small sample groups. This makes it difficult, if not impossible, to identify any side effects except those that are extremely common. It absolutely precludes the identification of rare side effects.

4. Many vaccines are studied in trials that do not have a proper placebo control. This makes it impossible to determine whether administering the vaccine is as safe as not administering it.

The last point is worth examining in greater detail, as properly controlled trials are the gold standard of medical research. Dr. Richard Moskowitz, MD has compiled data on placebos and on reports of adverse reactions from vaccine safety trials as of 2017, and his data is summarized in Table 3 below.[314] Dr. Moskowitz importantly distinguishes between the time period that the manufacturer used for the acceptance of "solicited" adverse reactions (those few diseases that the CDC has accepted as directly linked to specific vaccines, such as anaphylaxis) and "unsolicited" adverse reactions (a catch-all category for anything that patients or their parents notice and choose to report to the investigators in charge of the study). As with many other self-reporting processes, it is likely that the unsolicited reactions that are reported are significantly fewer than the actual reactions that occur among the patients in the study.

---

[314] Moskowitz R. *Vaccines: A Reappraisal*. New York: Skyhorse Publishing, 2017, p. 34-36.

All of the summarized trial data is published on the vaccine package inserts, and can be requested from doctors prior to any immunization or requested from the manufacturer.

| Vaccine | Brand and Manufacturer | Placebo Used | Solicited Adverse Reactions Accepted for: | Unsolicited Adverse Reactions Accepted for: |
|---|---|---|---|---|
| DTaP | Adacel, Sanofi-Pasteur | No controlled studies | 14 days | 6 months |
| Influenza, quadrivalent | Fluarix, GlaxoSmithKline | Sanofi-Pasteur influenza vaccine | 7 days | 21 days |
| Hepatitis B | Engerix, GlaxoSmithKline | No controlled studies | 4 days | No information available |
| Hepatitis B | Recombivax HB, Merck | No controlled studies | 5 days | No information available |
| Hib Conjugate | Hiberix, GlaxoSmithKline | Merck, Wyeth, or Sanofi-Pasteur Hib vaccine AND two other vaccines | 4 days | No information available |
| Hib Liquid Conjugate | Pedvax, Merck | lyophilized version of Hib vaccine and two other vaccines | 3 days | No information available |
| HPV | Cervarix, GlaxoSmithKline | Hepatitus A vaccine | 7 days | 30 days |
| HPV | Gardasil, Merck | 320 subjects: saline; 3,470 subjects: aluminum adjuvant | 14 days | |
| Measles, Mumps, and Rubella | MMRII, Merck | No safety studies | N/A | N/A |
| Pneumococcal, 23-valent | Pneumovax 23, Merck | 0.25% phenol | 5 days | No information available |
| Pneumococcal, 7-valent | Prevnar, Wyeth-Pfizer | No randomized controlled studies | 48 hours | 1 year |
| Polio, inactivated | IPV: IPOL, Sanofi-Pasteur | DTP vaccine | 48 hours | No information available |
| Rotavirus | Rotarix, GlaxoSmithKline | Unspecified placebo | 7 days | No information available |
| Rotavirus | RotaTeq, Merck | Unspecified placebo | 42 days | 42 days |
| Varicella (Chickenpox) | Varivax, Merck | Unspecified placebo | 42 days | No information available |
| Zoster (Shingles) | Zostavax, Merck | Unspecified placebo | 5 days | 5 years |

Table 3: Vaccine Trial Data on Placebo Use and Documentation of Adverse Side Effects

In addition to problems with placebos and a general lack of controlled studies, there is a tremendous issue with conflicts of interest in vaccine safety studies. The studies are generally funded by the vaccine manufacturers themselves, who control who has access to the data that is generated and how that data is ultimately reported. Questionable methods of modifying studies during or after data collection have been reported for many of these studies.[315,316]

Interpretation of study results can be another source of error even if the results are correctly reported. For example, many vaccine studies conclude that there is insufficient evidence to establish causal links between a given vaccine and a particular adverse reaction.[317] This result is then reported as a conclusion that the vaccine is "safe," rather than acknowledging that *the testing was insufficient to establish safety* for the same reason it was insufficient to establish harm.

## Vaccine Court: Another Ethical Issue

At the same time that the VAERS reporting system was created, Congress also created the Vaccine Injury Compensation Program (VICP) to allow parents of vaccine-injured children an avenue for redress of the damage done to their child, but at the same time to protect vaccine manufacturers from expensive lawsuits. This legal protection is unique to vaccine manufacturers (damages from all other drugs and medical devices are legally actionable through the normal court system) and was created in the mid-1980s to give manufacturers incentive to keep manufacturing vaccines after the DPT vaccine was found to be seriously damaging to those who received it.[318] Congress claimed that the purpose of the VICP was "to establish a no-fault program under which awards can be made to the vaccine-injured quickly, easily, and with certainty and generosity."[319] While the intention in creating the program may have been laudable, its execution has been fraught with problems from its inception.

Dr. Richard Moskowitz has outlined the necessary conditions for a claim to meet the VICP standards in his book *Vaccines: A Reappraisal*. He reports that a vaccine can only be claimed to have caused an adverse event if the following six conditions are met[320]:

1. The exact chronology of the event onset is known and can be correlated to the exact chronology of the vaccination.
2. The adverse event is one that has been previously described as a possible outcome for that particular vaccine.
3. There is a "biologically plausible" mechanism for the onset of the adverse event (that is recognized by the scientific community at large).

---

[315] Ibid, p. 39-41.

[316] Sears RW. *The Vaccine Book*. New York: Little, Brown and Company, 2011, p. 187-191.
For a fuller discussion of conflicts of interest in pharmaceutical research in general, please see: Goldacre B. *Bad Pharma*. New York: Faber and Faber, 2012.

[317] Institute of Medicine 2012. Adverse Effects of Vaccines: Evidence and Causality. Washington, DC: The National Academies Press. https://doi.org/10.17226/13164.

[318] Moskowitz, Richard MD. *Vaccines: A Reappraisal*. New York: Skyhorse Publishing, 2017, p. 122-123.

[319] H.R. Rep. No. 98-908 at 3(1986), reprinted in 1986 U.S.C.C.A.N.6344.
cf. Holland M, Conte L, Krakow R, Colin L. Unanswered Questions from the Vaccine Injury Compensation Program: A Review of Compensated Cases of Vaccine-Induced Brain Injury. Pace Environmental Law Review, 2011 Winter; 28(2): Citation 19.

[320] Moskowitz, Richard MD. *Vaccines: A Reappraisal*. New York: Skyhorse Publishing, 2017, p.124-125.

4. Laboratory tests can confirm an association between the vaccine and the adverse event.
5. A re-challenge of the system with the vaccine or a booster dose results in the same adverse event.
6. Controlled clinical trials confirm that this adverse event has been observed in safety tests for the vaccine.

As Dr. Moskowitz makes clear, there are a number of reasons why these stringent criteria rule out almost any adverse event from being accepted by the VICP. The onset of complex diseases, like the allergies and autoimmune conditions that were discussed above, is often complicated to sort out chronologically, particularly if parents were not on the alert to look for symptoms after a vaccination. The second and sixth point effectively restrict both the VICP and the VAERS system (which uses a strikingly similar table of reportable events[321]) from recognizing any new conditions that are associated with a vaccine – thus rendering them all but useless as any type of post-marketing safety surveillance for vaccine safety, which was part of the purpose of their creation. Many autoimmune conditions, as well as autism, are excluded by the "biologically plausible" requirement, as little is known about how these conditions actually develop and so little can be concluded about the biological mechanism of possible vaccine-induction of these conditions. Laboratory confirmation of a link between the event and the vaccine is not objectionable, but it is inconvenient and is rarely performed, and is often used after-the-fact to dismiss cases from adjudication by the VICP. Point five is both absurd and heinous; to re-challenge a child with something that they have already adversely reacted to is the height of medical malpractice, and implicitly discounts children who have died from the administration of a vaccine (since they are unavailable for re-challenge).[322]

From 1988 to July 2015, only 16,038 claims were filed in the VICP[323], as compared to 435,120 events reported to VAERS from July 1990 (the first available date on which searches could be run) through July 2015.[324] Even if only 10-15% of the events reported to VAERS are seriously adverse, as Dr. Sears claimed,[325] this means that at most 1/3 of all serious adverse reactions are even being addressed by the VICP. Of the 16,038 claims that were reported, only 4,150 claims were compensated – roughly ¼ of cases that come before the court, and at most 1/11 of all the serious adverse events that are reported. When we keep in mind that the VAERS system represents only 1-10% of actual reactions to vaccines, it is possible that less than 0.1% of all serious injuries from vaccination are actually compensated. This is an abysmally low rate for an organization that claims to make it easy and expedient for patients to pursue a legal recourse for this form of iatrogenic injury.

---

[321] Ibid, p. 129.
[322] Ibid, p. 125-127. All the relevant points I have made above are summarized from Dr. Moskowitz's arguments.
[323] Ibid, p. 136.
[324] CDC. The Vaccine Adverse Events Reporting System Results. Reports submitted July 1990 to July 2015. https://wonder.cdc.gov/controller/datarequest/D8;jsessionid=A096275431E3BE76010B6F1F8E2225B2 Accessed 28 Oct 2019.
[325] Sears RW. *The Vaccine Book*. New York: Little, Brown and Company, 2011, p. 192.

# The Coronavirus Response and Vaccination

*[I]f an intervention has any kind of suspected risk of harm, the burden of proof that it is not harmful must fall on those who recommend it.*
*-- Dr. Paul Thomas, MD[326]*

As of November 2020, it seems almost unreasonable to write at any length on the question of vaccination and not include a discussion of the possible vaccine for the 2019 coronavirus, SARS-CoV-2, that will likely be marketed to the public within months. Before beginning this part of the discussion, it should first be noted that the rush to publish papers on SARS-CoV-2, including those in journals that are not peer-reviewed, has led to a great deal of confusion about the nature of the virus and its actual impact on populations. There is also a great deal of confusion about COVID-19, a disease that is associated with SARS-CoV-2 infection. The confusion is furthered by the use of the terms "coronavirus" and "COVID-19" interchangeably, as well as the use of the term "coronavirus" to refer specifically to SARS-CoV-2 when there are seven coronaviruses that infect humans (four of which are common infections that cause mild cold-like symptoms).[327] The terminology used here may sound a bit unfamiliar, but in order not to add to the confusion, the coronaviruses under discussion will be referred to by their proper names: SARS-CoV-2 is the 2019 coronavirus, SARS-CoV began circulating in 2003 and is associated with severe acute respiratory syndrome (SARS), and MERS-CoV began circulating in 2012 and is associated with Middle East respiratory syndrome (MERS).

Questions about the nature of the SARS-CoV-2 virus and its effects are best resolved by time and by other authors who have more epidemiological experience. Even so, while there is much that is still unknown about the nature and effects of this *particular* virus, there has been a significant body of research in the past decade into developing vaccines for other coronaviruses – specifically those responsible for SARS and MERS – which should help inform our response to the vaccine candidates currently in development. There is also some historical evidence that suggests that mass-produced quick-turnaround vaccines are not likely to be safe. Regarding the latter point, a few recent examples of vaccines with extremely short turn-around times will be highly illustrative.

## Short Vaccine Development Timelines Result in Unsafe Vaccines

The HPV vaccine Gardasil® was fast-tracked by the FDA and approved in only six months.[328] The approval occurred before adequate safety trials were conducted on the vaccine; post-licensure safety trials were later done in India on a cohort of approximately 30,000 tribal girls, aged 9 to 15,

---

[326] Thomas P and Margulis J. *The Vaccine-Friendly Plan*. New York: Ballantine Books, 2016, p. 25.
[327] National Institutes of Health: National Institute of Allergy and Infectious Diseases. Coronaviruses. 19 May 2020. https://www.niaid.nih.gov/diseases-conditions/coronaviruses. Accessed 26 Sept 2020.
See also: Center for Disease Control. Human Coronaviruses. National Center for Immunization and Respiratory Diseases (NCIRD), Division of Viral Diseases. 15 Feb 2020. https://www.cdc.gov/coronavirus/types.html. Accessed 26 Sept 2020.
[328] Whitman H, Cajigal S. Timeline: 10 Years of the HPV Vaccine. Medscape. 05 Aug 2016. https://www.medscape.com/viewarticle/866964. Accessed 21 Sept 2020.

from two different locales.[329] Six deaths were reported in conjunction with the vaccinations.[330] Other serious adverse effects were detailed in an investigation done by a women's rights group in India:

> Many of the vaccinated girls continue to suffer from stomachaches, headaches, giddiness and exhaustion. There have been reports of early onset of menstruation, heavy bleeding and severe menstrual cramps, extreme mood swings, irritability, and uneasiness following the vaccination. No systematic follow up or monitoring has been carried out by the vaccine providers.[331]

Various news sources report the rate of adverse events in the trials that were conducted in India from 1 in 133 individuals[332] to 1 in 19[333]. While these rates are likely higher than they would have been in the US, due to the poverty and nutritional deficiencies of many of the tribal girls in the post-licensure study,[334] they are still alarming. From these reports alone, it seems quite clear that the vaccine should have been much more rigorously tested, and should not have been approved for mass administration so quickly. When these data are considered with the earlier discussion of the risks of infertility associated with the HPV vaccine, the case becomes even more clear that rapid vaccine development is imprudent and unsafe.

Another example of a vaccine that was rushed to production will lead us to similar conclusions, and this is the swine flu vaccine of 1976. The death of a young soldier at Fort Dix in February of 1976, followed by the isolation of a novel strain of swine flu circulating among the soldiers, prompted fears of a 1918-like pandemic.[335] The response of the United States government was to initiate a campaign to vaccinate every US citizen; legislation pushing for vaccines was signed into

---

[329] Kumar, KPN. Controversial vaccine studies: Why is Bill & Melinda Gates Foundation under fire from critics in India? Economic Times. 31 Aug 2014.
https://economictimes.indiatimes.com/industry/healthcare/biotech/healthcare/controversial-vaccine-studies-why-is-bill-melinda-gates-foundation-under-fire-from-critics-in-india/articleshow/41280050.cms?utm_source=contentofinterest&utm_medium=text&utm_campaign=cppst. Accessed 26 Sept 2020.
[330] Sama. Fact Finding of HPV Vaccine 'demonstration project' in Andhra Pradesh.
http://www.samawomenshealth.in/fact-finding-of-hpv-vaccine-demonstration-project-in-andhra-pradesh/ Accessed 26 Sept 2020.
[331] Ibid.
[332] Kumar, KPN. Controversial vaccine studies: Why is Bill & Melinda Gates Foundation under fire from critics in India? Economic Times. 31 Aug 2014.
https://economictimes.indiatimes.com/industry/healthcare/biotech/healthcare/controversial-vaccine-studies-why-is-bill-melinda-gates-foundation-under-fire-from-critics-in-india/articleshow/41280050.cms?utm_source=contentofinterest&utm_medium=text&utm_campaign=cppst. Accessed 26 Sept 2020.
[333] Mehta K, Bhanot N, Rao VR. Supreme Court Pulls Up Government Of India Over Licensing And Trials With "Cervical Cancer" Vaccines. Countercurrents. 07 Jan 2013.
https://www.countercurrents.org/mehta070113.htm. Accessed 26 Sept 2020.
[334] Sharma K. The Other Half: Uninformed Consent. The Hindu. 17 Apr 2010.
https://www.thehindu.com/opinion/columns/Kalpana_Sharma/The-Other-Half-Uninformed-consent/article16123576.ece Accessed 12 May 2020.
[335] Dehner G. WHO Knows Best? National and International Responses to Pandemic Threats and the "Lessons" of 1976. *Journal of the History of Medicine and Allied Sciences*, 2010, 64(4), 478-513.

effect in April.[336]   Vaccinations began on October 1st, [337] despite the fact that there were no confirmed cases of swine flu – worldwide – beyond the handful at Fort Dix.[338]   Initial studies on candidate vaccines were promising enough for the campaign to move forward.   However, a different vaccine formulation was used during the campaign from the one that had actually been field tested, according to the admission of Dr. David Sencer (then head of the CDC); this new formulation had not been tested in clinical trials.[339]   Dr. Michael Hatwick, who advised the CDC on safety issues with the 1976 campaign, had notified that office of the potential for neurological damage associated with the vaccine, but his warnings went unheeded.[340]

The campaign was an unmitigated disaster:

> The Swine Flu Program was marred by a series of logistical problems ranging from the production of the wrong vaccine strain to a confrontation over liability protection to a temporal connection of the vaccine and a cluster of deaths among an elderly population in Pittsburgh.   The most damning charge against the vaccination program was that the shots were correlated with an increase in the number of patients diagnosed with an obscure neurological disease known as Guillain–Barre´ syndrome [GBS].   The program was halted when the statistical increase was detected, but ultimately the New York Times labeled the program a "fiasco" because the feared pandemic never appeared.[341]

A *60 Minutes* documentary exposing the problems with the vaccine campaign reported that 46 million Americans received the shot, and 4,000 claimed damages in a lawsuit filed against the federal government. [342]   Vaccine manufacturers themselves were protected from liability, as they had issued an ultimatum to legislators for indemnity to damages in the event the vaccine proved to have adverse side effects.[343]   Two thirds of the claimants' cases were for neurological damage, many of them for GBS.   The CDC still acknowledges GBS is a risk associated with the influenza vaccine as of 2020, though their website tries to downplay the seriousness of this issue.[344]   The risk of developing GBS from the fast-produced shot of 1976 was ten times greater than the seasonal flu shot.[345]

---

[336] Eschner K. The Long Shadow of the 1976 Swine Flu Vaccine 'Fiasco'. Smithsonian Magazine. 6 Feb 2017. https://www.smithsonianmag.com/smart-news/long-shadow-1976-swine-flu-vaccine-fiasco-180961994/ Accessed 26 Sept 2020.

[337] Ibid.

[338] Wallace M. The Swine Flu Fraud of 1976. *60 Minutes*. Available on https://www.youtube.com/watch?v=Ydx_ok6gyiY Accessed 26 May 2020.

[339] Ibid.

[340] Ibid.

[341] Dehner G. WHO Knows Best? National and International Responses to Pandemic Threats and the "Lessons" of 1976. *Journal of the History of Medicine and Allied Sciences*, 2010, 64(4), 478-513.

[342] Wallace M. The Swine Flu Fraud of 1976. *60 Minutes*. Available on https://www.youtube.com/watch?v=Ydx_ok6gyiY Accessed 26 May 2020.

[343] Sencer DJ, Millar JD. Reflections on the 1976 Swine Flu Vaccination Program. *Emerging Infectious Diseases*, 2006 Jan, 12(1), 29-33.

[344] Center for Disease Control. Guillain-Barré Syndrome and Vaccines. 14 Aug 2020. https://www.cdc.gov/vaccinesafety/concerns/guillain-barre-syndrome.html#:~:text=When%20there%20has%20been%20an,the%20flu%20than%20after%20vaccination. Accessed 26 Sept 2020.

[345] Ibid.

Part of the tragedy of these vaccine injuries is that the expected epidemic never materialized. Interestingly, attempts were made to combat two earlier influenza pandemics via vaccination, in 1957 and 1968. In both cases, the infections peaked before the vaccines could be developed and administered to a sufficient number of individuals.[346] We may be observing a similar situation with the SARS-CoV-2 coronavirus; as has routinely been documented, predictions about viral epidemics are about as reliable as the weather forecast, and those who are predicting a deadly resurgence of coronavirus infections in the fall of 2020 may be as misguided as the harbingers of the 1976 pandemic.

## Coronavirus Vaccines: 17 Years of Failed Attempts

In addition to general concerns about the rush of the vaccine to production, there is ample evidence that it may be particularly difficult to develop vaccines against members of the virus group to which the SARS-CoV-2 coronavirus belongs.

SARS was the first disease of international concern to be caused by a coronavirus. The virus spread from China in 2002, with a peak number of cases in 2003 (at which point SARS was labeled a pandemic).[347] The first candidate for a vaccine against SARS-CoV began clinical trials in China in 2005.[348] Fifteen years later, we are still without a safe and effective coronavirus vaccine for SARS-CoV. This point is simple, but it cannot be overlooked – it verges on insanity to think that a safe and effective vaccine can be developed for SARS-CoV-2 in less than a year when researchers have met with a decade and a half of failure working on vaccine candidates for a very similar virus.

Neither do we have a vaccine for MERS-CoV, another coronavirus that drew international attention after being isolated from a Saudi Arabian male who died of pneumonia in 2012.[349] SARS has a case fatality rate of approximately 10%, while MERS has a case fatality of approximately 34%.[350] The high case fatality rates of these viruses have certainly fueled a serious research and development plan for vaccine candidates for both SARS and MERS: a quick search on PubMed for academic articles relating to the development of vaccine candidates for these coronaviruses yields over 6,400 results from the last seventeen years.[351]

In that time period, researchers have learned a number of valuable lessons about the nature of developing vaccines against coronaviruses. The use of the whole virus in an inactivated virus vaccine (which is generally considered the safest type of vaccine to develop on a short-term/large-

---

[346] Dehner G. WHO Knows Best? National and International Responses to Pandemic Threats and the "Lessons" of 1976. *Journal of the History of Medicine and Allied Sciences*, 2010, 64(4), 478-513.

[347] Song Z, Xu Y, Bao L, et al. From SARS to MERS, Thrusting Coronaviruses into the Spotlight. *Viruses*. 2019 Jan 14;11(1):59. doi: 10.3390/v11010059.

[348] Jiang S, He Y, Liu S. SARS vaccine development. *Emerg Infect Dis*. 2005;11(7):1016-1020. doi:10.3201/1107.050219.

[349] Song Z, Xu Y, Bao L, et al. From SARS to MERS, Thrusting Coronaviruses into the Spotlight. *Viruses*. 2019 Jan 14;11(1):59. doi: 10.3390/v11010059.

[350] Hewings-Martin Y. How do SARS and MERS compare with COVID-19? *Medical News Today*. 10 Apr 2020. https://www.medicalnewstoday.com/articles/how-do-sars-and-mers-compare-with-covid-19 Accessed 27 Sept 2020.

[351] Searches for "SARS vaccine" and "MERS vaccine" on https://pubmed.ncbi.nlm.nih.gov/

scale basis)[352] produced an unexpected result: a skewing of the immune response towards activation of a particular type of T cells, T helper 2 ($T_h2$).[353] This type of response can result in elevated levels of two types of innate immune cells in the blood (eosinophils, which are associated with allergies, and neutrophils); this elevation, in turn, drives an inflammatory response that can significantly damage the body. Eosinophils in particular can cause organ damage in the skin, heart, lungs, digestive tract, and nervous system when their levels are elevated.[354] Researchers found that vaccinating ferrets and primates with the inactivated SARS-CoV vaccine candidates resulted in inflammatory pathology (disease) in the vaccinated animals, rather than effective clearance of the virus.[355] One particular inactivated vaccine caused eosinophil levels in the lungs to rise significantly in vaccinated animals; this occurred after they had been challenged (infected) with the SARS-CoV virus. This eosinophilic infiltration may also have promoted allergic responses in some of the older animals.[356]

In addition, some researchers found that the SARS-CoV vaccines actually enhanced the virulence of the disease when the test subjects were later challenged with an infection. This was mediated through antibodies to a particular segment to the SARS-CoV spike protein.[357] Concerns regarding this "antibody dependent enhancement," as it has been called, were raised in the Proceedings of the National Academy of Sciences (PNAS) as early as April of 2020, but were considered less important than the $T_h2$ cell pathology just described.[358]

It is also possible that the overall level of circulating antibody in the blood can determine whether a vaccine is protective against a disease or instead actually enhances the disease pathology. Lower levels of circulating SARS-CoV antibody, comparable to those likely to be produced during a mass vaccination campaign of the general population, were associated with increased infection by the virus.[359]

Authors in *Nature Reviews*, a prestigious peer-reviewed journal, noted these additional areas of concern about SARS-CoV vaccines: [360]

---

[352] Jiang S, He Y, Liu S. SARS vaccine development. *Emerg Infect Dis*. 2005;11(7):1016-1020. doi:10.3201/1107.050219.

[353] Graham RL, Donaldson EF, Ralph SB. A decade after SARS: Strategies for controlling emerging coronaviruses. *Nature Reviews*. 2013 Dec, 11. doi: 10.1038/nrmicro3143

[354] Tefferi A. Blood eosinophilia: a new paradigm in disease classification, diagnosis, and treatment. *Mayo Clin Proc*. 2005; 80:75.

[355] Graham RL, Donaldson EF, Ralph SB. A decade after SARS: Strategies for controlling emerging coronaviruses. *Nature Reviews*. 2013 Dec, 11. doi: 10.1038/nrmicro3143

[356] Bolles M, et al. A double-inactivated severe acute respiratory syndrome coronavirus vaccine provides incomplete protection in mice and induces increased eosinophilic proinflammatory pulmonary response upon challenge. *J Virol*. 2011, 85: 12201-12215.

[357] Wang Q, Zhang L, Kuwahara K, et al. Immunodominant SARS Coronavirus Epitopes in Humans Elicited both Enhancing and Neutralizing Effects on Infection in Non-human Primates. *ACS Infect Dis*. 2016, 2: 361-376.

[358] Peeples L. News Feature: Avoiding pitfalls in the pursuit of a COVID-19 vaccine. *PNAS* 2020 Apr 17; 117(15): 8218-8221.

[359] Luo F, et al. Evaluation of Antibody-Dependent Enhancement of SARS-CoV Infection in Rhesus Macaques Immunized with an Inactivated SARS-CoV Vaccine. *Virologica Sinica*. 2018, 33: 201-2-4.

[360] Graham RL, Donaldson EF, Ralph SB. A decade after SARS: Strategies for controlling emerging coronaviruses. *Nature Reviews*. 2013 Dec, 11. doi: 10.1038/nrmicro3143

- Animal models used for vaccine development are insufficient to study the kind of severe clinical response that is seen in humans who develop SARS. Thus, a candidate that is effective in animals may not be effective in humans, and vice versa.
- There is a poor response to the majority of vaccine candidates among the most vulnerable populations, those 65 years and older.
- Live attenuated vaccines carried a possibility of the vaccine strain mutating back to wild-type and becoming fully infective, which means that these vaccines could actually cause the person to contract the disease. This type of vaccine may also result in recombination with naturally circulating virus, which could generate a new strain of coronavirus with unknown infectivity. This second scenario is particularly troubling.

In addition to inactivated and live virus vaccines, there are a number of novel vaccine modalities that are being explored in the attempt to develop a vaccine both for SARS-CoV and SARS-CoV-2. Viral vector vaccines, in which a non-pathogenic virus is engineered to carry DNA and/or proteins from a pathogenic virus, are among these novel platforms. When vaccines to SARS-CoV were developed using these vectors, protection against infection appeared to be incomplete, particularly in older individuals.[361] DNA vaccine candidates, which are also among the current favorites for SARS-CoV-2 development, have not been tested using lethal-challenge models for other coronavirus vaccines, so there is limited to no data on how protective this type of vaccine might be in the event of a pandemic.[362]

Even Pfizer, which claimed on November 18, 2020, to be producing a vaccine that is 95% effective,[363] had this to say in the fine print of their press release:

> This release contains forward-looking information about Pfizer's efforts to combat COVID-19, the collaboration between BioNTech and Pfizer to develop a potential COVID-19 vaccine, the BNT162 mRNA vaccine program, and modRNA candidate BNT162b2 (including qualitative assessments of available data, potential benefits, expectations for clinical trials, anticipated timing of regulatory submissions and anticipated manufacturing, distribution and supply), that involves substantial risks and uncertainties that could cause actual results to differ materially from those expressed or implied by such statements. Risks and uncertainties include, among other things, the uncertainties inherent in research and development, including the ability to meet anticipated clinical endpoints, commencement and/or completion dates for clinical trials, regulatory submission dates, regulatory approval dates and/or launch dates, as well as risks associated with clinical data (including the Phase 3 data that is the subject of this release), including the possibility of unfavorable new preclinical or clinical trial data and further analyses of existing preclinical or clinical trial data; the ability to produce comparable clinical or other results, including the rate of vaccine effectiveness and safety and tolerability profile observed to date, in additional analyses of the Phase 3 trial or in larger, more diverse populations upon commercialization; the risk that clinical trial data are subject to differing interpretations

[361] Ibid.
[362] Ibid.
[363] Pfizer. Pfizer and Biontech conclude phase-3 study of COVID-19 vaccine candidate, meeting all primary efficacy endpoints. 18 Nov 2020. https://www.pfizer.com/news/press-release/press-release-detail/pfizer-and-biontech-conclude-phase-3-study-covid-19-vaccine Accessed 18 Nov 2020.

and assessments, including during the peer review/publication process, in the scientific community generally, and by regulatory authorities; whether and when data from the BNT162 mRNA vaccine program will be published in scientific journal publications and, if so, when and with what modifications; whether regulatory authorities will be satisfied with the design of and results from these and any future preclinical and clinical studies; whether and when any biologics license and/or emergency use authorization applications may be filed in any jurisdictions for BNT162b2 or any other potential vaccine candidates; whether and when any such applications may be approved by regulatory authorities, which will depend on myriad factors, including making a determination as to whether the vaccine candidate's benefits outweigh its known risks and determination of the vaccine candidate's efficacy and, if approved, whether it will be commercially successful; decisions by regulatory authorities impacting labeling, manufacturing processes, safety and/or other matters that could affect the availability or commercial potential of a vaccine, including development of products or therapies by other companies; disruptions in the relationships between us and our collaboration partners or third-party suppliers; risks related to the availability of raw materials to manufacture a vaccine; challenges related to our vaccine candidate's ultra-low temperature formulation and attendant storage, distribution and administration requirements, including risks related to handling after delivery by Pfizer; the risk that we may not be able to successfully develop non-frozen formulations; the risk that we may not be able to create or scale up manufacturing capacity on a timely basis or have access to logistics or supply channels commensurate with global demand for any potential approved vaccine, which would negatively impact our ability to supply the estimated numbers of doses of our vaccine candidate within the projected time periods indicated; whether and when additional supply agreements will be reached; uncertainties regarding the ability to obtain recommendations from vaccine technical committees and other public health authorities and uncertainties regarding the commercial impact of any such recommendations; uncertainties regarding the impact of COVID-19 on Pfizer's business, operations and financial results; and competitive developments.[364]

It should be noted that at the time of this release, Pfizer's data has not been peer-reviewed or published, little to nothing is known about the composition of their trial groups (particularly about effectiveness in older adults), and – most damning of all – the data analysis was conducted using a paltry 170 cases of COVID-19 diagnoses (approximately).[365] In addition, the trial evidences a conspicuous lack of testing for actual SARS-CoV-2 infection, raising the question of whether vaccinated individuals could still contract and be carriers of the disease.[366] It would seem that sanguine predictions of success are overblown, and the real science of coronavirus vaccine development is being largely ignored. Despite the optimism of certain vaccine proponents, there is little to no likelihood of a SARS-CoV-2 vaccine being produced in less than a year that is both effective in preventing infection by the virus and safe to administer without egregious side effects.

---

[364] Ibid.

[365] Ibid.

[366] Mercola, JD. First COVID-19 Vaccine 90% Effective? 18 Nov 2020. www.articles.mercola.com/sites/articles/archive/2020/11/18/first-covid-19-vaccine-90-percent-effective.aspx Accessed 18 Nov 2020.

# Where Can We Go from Here?

*What an act of insanity it would be to implant the infective products of undefined disease into the bodies of eight thousand healthy children in order to prevent the possible development of a very few mild cases of small-pox! Could absurdity go further than this?*
*-- Dr. J.W. Hodge, 1911[367]*

When I began the research for this paper, I was still a vaccine advocate. I devoted my graduate studies to developing ethical alternatives to aborted fetal vaccines, to remove what I saw as the most negative consequence of vaccination; I sought to reform the practice, not reject it. I knew some vaccines (like HPV and influenza vaccines) were dangerous, but I did not have the remotest inkling of the depth of the problem that I have outlined in this short work. I had no idea that the whole paradigm of safety and efficacy that I had accepted so readily was built upon such an imprecise and pseudo-scientific basis, that vaccination had always been opposed by people who were quite rational in their opposition, or that there were so many documented cases of harm and such reasonable biological mechanisms proposed to explain them. As the import of all of this began to dawn on me, my first question was the last question I will address in this treatise – if vaccines are truly harmful, where do we go from here? What reasonable alternatives are open to us?

Choosing to vaccinate and choosing not to vaccinate both carry consequences, and they must be weighed by individual families, in light of the information available about risks and benefits.

## Will the World be at Risk if We Do Not Vaccinate?

As we have seen, we will face challenges of new and emerging pathogens regardless of whether populations are vaccinated or not. In fact, vaccination in some cases has sped up the process of emerging infections by providing new diseases with a niche in which to propagate. This has created additional problems with infectious diseases, and will continue to create problems as long as mass vaccination is continued.

It must be remembered that there are no risk-free options in this life after the Fall of Adam. If we stop vaccination for a disease wholesale, we are likely to see at least a temporary resurgence of the disease, since the vaccines have effectively destroyed real herd immunity. However, a new wave of a "vaccine preventable" disease will almost certainly never reach the levels of mortality observed at the turn of the 20th century, due to improved sanitation and other public health measures. Some vaccine advocates claim that to abandon mass vaccination would result in an apocalyptic scenario of disease and death; however, there is more than enough established scientific evidence to suggest that the opposite may actually be true. If normal childhood pathogens were allowed to circulate again in the population, it is likely that natural "priming" of the immune systems of children would lessen the likelihood of them developing cancer and other long-term chronic conditions. In addition, the natural "boosting" effect of circulating pathogens would protect adults from illnesses such as shingles and rubella.

---

[367] As quoted in Humphries S and Bystrianyk R. *Dissolving Illusions.* Printed by author. 2015, p. 124.

## *What about Rabies? And Other Worst Case Scenarios*

You might say that the above attitude is fine for things like chickenpox – but what about diseases that have extremely high fatality rates, like rabies or tetanus? What are the risks and benefits for using vaccines in these cases?

There are approximately two deaths from rabies per year in the United States,[368] and approximately 30,000-60,000 people receive treatment for possible rabies exposure.[369] Part of this treatment is the use of a rabies vaccine. The vaccine works in the same way as other vaccines – it is an inactivated form of the rabies virus that is administered in the shoulder muscle. The difference is that it is usually given *therapeutically* rather than *prophylactically*; that is, the vaccine is given *after* actual exposure is suspected, rather than *before* there is any chance of encountering the disease (as is done with the majority of vaccines). Most vaccines cannot be administered therapeutically, and will worsen the disease progression if administered after exposure to the pathogen. However, because the rabies virus has such a long incubation period, the exposure to the inactivated virus in the vaccine will initiate the body's immune response early enough to prevent a full-blown rabies infection (from which there is no cure).[370] The rabies vaccine does have a number of common adverse side effects (including soreness, headaches, nausea, and vomiting)[371] but the rabies virus is almost inevitably fatal. In this case, using the vaccine as a therapeutic option makes a great deal of sense; even using it prophylactically makes a great deal of sense when one's job involves a great deal of exposure to wild animals. However, one should be careful to ensure that the form of the vaccine given is ethical – Imovax, by Sanofi-Pasteur, is produced in the MRC-5 aborted fetal cell line.[372] Vaccinees can request RabAvert by GlaxoSmithKline as an ethical alternative.[373]

The tetanus vaccine is recommended by the CDC both prophylactically and therapeutically.[374] The vaccine is a toxoid vaccine, so it does not result in an immune response that clears the pathogen more quickly, but rather an immune response that neutralizes the toxin produced by the pathogen (which can severely damage the nervous system). Though tetanus has a similarly long incubation period to rabies, an initial search of the literature did not produce any evidence that suggested the tetanus vaccine would have a similar effect to the rabies vaccine if used therapeutically. Clinical treatment also includes use of antibodies (immunoglobulin injections),[375] so it is unclear whether recovery in patients is due to the use of the vaccine or to other therapeutic agents. The tetanus vaccine is always administered either in combination with the diphtheria vaccine (DT) or with

---

[368] Pieracci EG, Pearson CM, Wallace RM, et al. Vital Signs: Trends in Human Rabies Deaths and Exposures - United States, 1938-2018. MMWR Morb Mortal Wkly Rep. 2019;68(23):524-528. Published 2019 Jun 14. doi:10.15585/mmwr.mm6823e1

[369] CDC. Human Rabies. 6 Apr 2020. https://www.cdc.gov/rabies/location/usa/surveillance/human_rabies.html. Accessed 31 May 2020.

[370] Offit, PA. A Look at Each Vaccine: Rabies Vaccine. Children's Hospital of Philadelphia. 20 July 2020. https://www.chop.edu/centers-programs/vaccine-education-center/vaccine-details/rabies-vaccine. Accessed 03 Oct 2020.

[371] Ibid.

[372] Children of God for Life. Aborted Fetal Cell Line Products for USA & Canada – And Ethical Alternatives. Jun 2020. https://cogforlife.org/wp-content/uploads/vaccineListOrigFormat.pdf. Accessed 03 Oct 2020.

[373] Ibid.

[374] CDC. Tetanus: For Clinicians. 23 Jan 2020. https://www.cdc.gov/tetanus/clinicians.html. Accessed 03 Oct 2020.

[375] Ibid.

both the diphtheria and pertussis vaccines (DTaP and Tdap, and formerly DPT). The DTaP and Tdap vaccines have an acknowledged severe adverse reaction rate of 1 in 10,000 vaccinees[376]; this rate may be much higher given the inaccuracies in the VAERS reporting system discussed earlier. In contrast, the chance of an individual contracting tetanus is approximately 1 in 128,000 in the United States, and the chance dying from tetanus is approximately 1 in 641,000.[377] In this case, the relative risk associated with receiving either the DTaP or the Tdap is significantly higher than the risk of contracting the disease.

For both rabies and tetanus, good judgement should be used on the part of individuals assessing their relative risk based on occupation and other factors. Neither disease, in my opinion, warrants a sufficient justification for continuing wholesale mass vaccination policies.

## Good Health – The Best Prophylaxis

Rather than relying on a vaccine jab to protect one from disease, individuals would be much better served if greater attention were given to maintaining a healthy immune system that could do its God-given work. Ultimately, we must also reject the evolutionary paradigm of the body as a sum of randomly mutated parts, and the idea that man's intelligence is necessary to intervene and "fix" the body's immune system, lest it be unable to deal with the threats to which we are constantly exposed by the world around us. The truths that we confess as members of the Catholic faith include the idea that the world – and our bodies – are damaged by the Fall, but they are not wholly corrupt. Man's body was created perfect in the beginning, and it was designed to run optimally. The body has a marvelous capacity to heal and repair itself, and it has been carrying out this function since the creation of man. While this capacity has diminished the further we are removed from the perfection of Adam, it is still sufficient for survival in most circumstances – provided that we are good stewards of what we have been given.

Health in general has much more to do with nutrition, sanitation, and physical exertion than it has to do with any medicines available – now or in the future. And health is profoundly individual, as recent studies on the microbiome suggest and our own experiences often confirm – it cannot be reduced to a one-size-fits-all program that ignores real contraindications and expects that all bodies (with their varying genetic makeup and accumulated differences from varied environmental exposures) will react in the same way to the same interventions. Despite all the research available about both modern and alternative healthcare, no single course of action can be universally recommended as *the* method for achieving good health without vaccination, due to the incredible variance in human bodies with their different predispositions and levels of immune reactivity. However, there are some general guidelines that the reader may find helpful:

- Eat whole foods. It is almost axiomatic in the field of nutrition today that avoiding processed foods will improve health, and this is considered to be the primary reason for the

---

[376] Offit, P. A Look at Each Vaccine: Diphtheria, Tetanus, and Pertussis Vaccines. Children's Hospital of Philadelphia. 07 Apr 2020. https://www.chop.edu/centers-programs/vaccine-education-center/vaccine-details/diphtheria-tetanus-and-pertussis-vaccines Accessed 03 Oct 2020.

[377] Calculations based on a birth rate of approximately 3,850,000 children per year, a tetanus infection rate of 30 persons per year, and a fatality rate of 10-20%.
See: CDC. Tetanus: For Clinicians. 23 Jan 2020. https://www.cdc.gov/tetanus/clinicians.html. Accessed 03 Oct 2020.

wholesomeness of a wide variety of traditional diets.[378]  Which foods are recommended will vary depending on which authors you read – some recommend diets that are high in fat, while others recommend diets that are high in vegetables, etc, etc.  The specific foods you choose to consume will vary depending on your culture, your own health condition, and your family's needs.  Nevertheless, the general principle is universally applicable – eat food in as close to its naturally-produced state as possible.  This includes avoiding foods that are heavily processed, genetically modified, or treated with exogenous chemicals such as antibiotics, pesticides, and hormones.

- Exercise when you are well, and rest when you are not.  There is a tremendous body of evidence that supports the idea that our bodies were made to move (not to sit) and it is also almost axiomatic that the average American lifestyle is too sedentary for the body to be as healthy as it would otherwise be.  However, there is coupled with this a curious excess of activity – individuals often have excessively busy lives that keep them on the job for many extra hours each week, or running from one scheduled event to another with no chance to pause in between.  This flurry of activity is rarely interrupted for something like a head cold, when the best medicine for most infections is often just to keep the body still and let the immune system perform its normal functions without the body being exhausted by its normal level of activity.  When you feel sick and want to sit around or sleep all day, your body is actually indicating to you that this would be quite helpful to your recovery.

- Supplement with vitamins and minerals when necessary.  This is an area where health advice must be quite individualized – not all persons share the same deficiencies, and not all persons have the same nutritional and mineral requirements.  What the body needs can vary depending on age, sex, activity level, preexisting health conditions, and many other factors.  In some cases, it may be helpful to have blood tests to determine specific deficiencies.  It is also important to research what chemical form of particular vitamins and minerals are most bioavailable, as not all forms can be used equally well in the body.

One final caution must be given for the benefit of readers who may be tempted to abandon modern medicine wholesale after reading this work and seek healthcare solely from alternative providers.  A number of common "alternative health" practices can be apparently effective, but this does not necessarily mean that they are safe for Catholics to use.  Many of these practices – such as acupuncture, applied kinesiology, homeopathy, and yoga – have deep roots in the occult.  There are two basic guidelines that can be used to determine whether an alternative health practice is safe and legitimate for Catholics[379]:

1. Is there a legitimate biological basis for the practice?
2. Is there significant occult influence in the history or development of the practice?

The answer to the first question should be "yes."  If the practice does not have a clear biological mechanism of action, it is likely that it is supposed to act through some sort of vital energy in the body; this type of practice is clearly occult and should be avoided (and confessed even if

---

[378] Shanahan C, Shanahan L. *Deep Nutrition: Why Your Genes Need Traditional Food*. Lawai, HI: Big Box Books, 2009, p. i-iv.
[379] Private communication with Fr. Chad Ripperger.

unintentionally practiced). Sometimes scientific studies can be helpful to determine the legitimacy of a treatment, but the reader should be careful to look for studies that have a large number of subjects and have clear control groups that do not receive the treatment.

The answer to the second question should be "no." While there are some practices that have occult roots that can be used by practitioners without any immediate formal cooperation with evil, occult influence often still remains in the way that the practices are taught and disseminated. Prudence is necessary here, but occult roots should give pause to a Catholic who wishes to practice the faith seriously.

Note that not all alternative health practices are occult in nature – some are based on sound biological principles, and there are a number of time-honored herbal remedies that are both effective and spiritually safe.*

This leads to the final recommendation for good health: because the soul is the form of the body, the health of our souls undoubtedly affects the health of our bodies. It is quite true that God allows some souls to suffer much in their body while still being in a state of grace, but it should also be kept in mind that one of the best ways to live well is to live according to natural law and to devote sufficient attention to one's spiritual life so as to always remain in the state of grace.

## In Closing

God's works are wonderful beyond our imagining, and the human body is undoubtedly one of His greatest works. With that in mind, I would like to conclude this brief study of vaccination by acknowledging how little we really understand about the working of the divinely-designed immune system and how salutary it would be for mankind if medical researchers devoted less time to developing vaccines and more time to studying natural immunity. We should learn how to optimize this marvelous system, instead of trying to tinker with it or bypass it in ways that compromise the health of the whole body for the sake of gaining a dubious advantage in the fight against a specific infectious disease.

When scientific and medical researchers approach the immune system within the Creation-Providence framework, they will no longer presume that the immune system is the product of millions of years of random mutation and natural selection, but a system intentionally fashioned by the Creator to keep the human body in a state of good health. Abandonment of the evolutionary hypothesis will allow researchers to discard the bankrupt notion of the body as a collection of disparate parts that are somewhat defective and must be modified to achieve their proper function, and to search for the causes of illness in dietary, genetic, physiological, psychological, spiritual, or environmental factors. This, in turn, will focus their attention on trying to discover much more thoroughly how the divinely-designed immune system actually works so that medical practitioners can help to optimize its God-given efficiency rather than bypassing it in ways that seriously

---

* A notable exception to this is Bach Flower Remedies, which are "potentized" similarly to homeopathic remedies and are New Age in nature.
     The curious reader can investigate Fr. James Manjackal's excellent collection of articles on homeopathy for additional information on this topic: http://www.jmanjackal.net/eng/enghomeo.htm

weaken the whole system.  When this paradigm shift happens, we will see a dramatic recovery of health on a national and global scale.

# Index